Aflatoxins - Occurrence, Detection and Novel Detoxification Strategies

Edited by Jean Claude Assaf

Published in London, United Kingdom

Aflatoxins - Occurrence, Detection and Novel Detoxification Strategies
http://dx.doi.org/10.5772/intechopen.100872
Edited by Jean Claude Assaf

Contributors
Anup Ramdas Kodape, Chikkarasanahalli Shivegowda Vivek Babu, Ashika Raveendran, Bismark Dabuo, Emmanuella Wesome Avogo, Gabriel Owusu Koomson, Maxwell Akantabila, Daniel Ayendo Gbati, Surya Kanta Mishra, Bijaya Kumar Swain, Lukman Bola Abdulra'Uf, Kikelomo Elizabeth Ayeni, Abibat Monisola Junaid, Aisha Ishaq, Abdulraahman Ibraheem, Muinat Aliu, Abubakar Lawal, Guan Huat Tan, Mohamed Mutocheluh, Patrick Williams Narkwa, Godfrey Z. Magoke, Robyn G. Alders, Mark Krockenberger, Wayne L. Bryden, Jean Claude Assaf, Rouaa Daou, André El Khoury

First published in London, United Kingdom, 2022 by IntechOpen
IntechOpen is the global imprint of INTECHOPEN LIMITED, registered in England and Wales, registration number: 11086078, 5 Princes Gate Court, London, SW7 2QJ, United Kingdom

British Library Cataloguing-in-Publication Data
A catalogue record for this book is available from the British Library

Additional hard and PDF copies can be obtained from orders@intechopen.com

Aflatoxins - Occurrence, Detection and Novel Detoxification Strategies
Edited by Jean Claude Assaf
p. cm.
Print ISBN 978-1-80356-884-3
Online ISBN 978-1-80356-885-0
eBook (PDF) ISBN 978-1-80356-886-7

Meet the editor

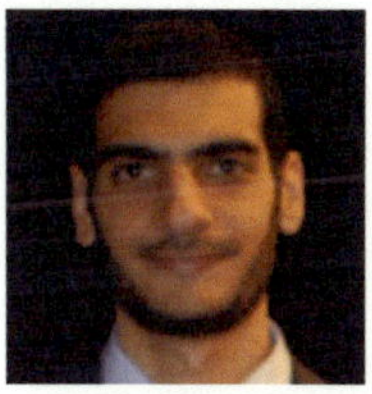

Dr. Jean-Claude Assaf is a lecturer at the Faculty of Sciences and the Faculty of Engineering at Saint Joseph University, and Lebanese University. He has won several national and international awards including the Lebanese Industrial Research Achievements (LIRA) award. His expertise lies in mycology and microbiology, particularly mycotoxins detoxification, lactic acid bacteria, and biofilms. Dr. Assaf is the owner of different industrial patents related to mycotoxins detoxification using novel adsorbents and machines. He has edited two books and edited, reviewed, and published numerous articles in international peer-reviewed journals.

Contents

Preface

The contamination of food and feed by aflatoxins remains a worldwide concern and a global threat to humans and animals. Accordingly, it can occur at any level from pre- to post-harvest, including transportation and storage. Aflatoxins are known to be highly carcinogenic, hence the consumption of aflatoxin-contaminated food can affect the liver, immune system, and other body functions. The occurrence of aflatoxin usually increases in warm and humid climates where different commodities such as maize, dried fruits, and spices as well as meat products and milk are at high contamination risk. There exist numerous detection methods for aflatoxins, such as liquid chromatography, infrared imaging, fluorescence imaging, and enzyme-linked immunosorbent assay (ELISA). Thus, by improving or creating new detection methods, highly accurate results can be generated in a short-term manner. Due to their harmful effect, the detoxification of aflatoxins remains a crucial industrial problem. This detoxification can be conducted using diverse chemical, physical, and biological methods. First, the physical methods rely on using a different kinds of adsorbents to control food or feed contamination. Second, the use of chemical substances for detoxification may also be an option when using safe chemicals. Nevertheless, biological detoxification using lactic acid bacteria, yeast, and other non-pathogenic microorganisms is progressively becoming a suitable detoxification approach due to its high specificity and safety profile. The discovery of new promising agents and technologies for aflatoxin detoxification is imperative and may lead to the elimination of the danger caused by these toxic metabolites.

Jean Claude Assaf
Saint Joseph University and Lebanese University,
Beirut, Lebanon

Chapter 1

Aflatoxins in the Era of Climate Change: The Mediterranean Experience

Rouaa Daou, Jean Claude Assaf and André El Khoury

Abstract

Aspergilluss sp. is a fungi that attack crops on the field or during storage. Generally, those fungi are most frequent in tropical and subtropical regions where environmental factors characterized by high humidity and temperatures are favorable for their production. Aflatoxins are produced as their secondary metabolites including aflatoxin B_1. Aflatoxins have been classified as carcinogenic to human by the International Agency for Research on Cancer due to their profound health effects, mainly, hepatocarcinogenicity. Hence, they contaminate a large share of the global food chain. Traditionally, aflatoxin contamination was not frequent in temperate regions such as the Mediterranean, however, with climate change patterns including elevated temperatures, increased humidity, and increased droughts, a shift in fungal attack patterns is expected in such areas in a way that favors *Aspergillus* sp. infestation and aflatoxin contamination. Therefore, with increased global warming more aflatoxin contamination is expected in the Mediterranean basin, specifically, the Sothern European countries.

Keywords: aflatoxins, climate change, Mediterranean

1. Introduction

1.1 Aflatoxins

Aflatoxins (AFs) are a group of mycotoxins produced by *Aspergillus* species mainly by *A. flavus* and *A. parasiticus* [1] and to a lesser extent, by *A. bombycis*, *A. ochraceoroseus*, *A. nomius*, and *A. pseudotamari* [2]. Eighteen AFs have been identified so far, but the ones with major significance are aflatoxin B_1 (AFB1), aflatoxin B_2, aflatoxin G_1, aflatoxin G_2, aflatoxin M_1, and aflatoxin M_2 [1, 3]. AFs are difuranocoumarin molecules that are produced by the polyketide pathway of fungi. Molecular differences among AF groups exist; for example, the B-aflatoxins exhibit a cyclopentane ring while the G-aflatoxins have a lactone ring (**Figure 1**) [3]. In addition to that, B-aflatoxins display blue fluorescence under ultraviolet light, while G-aflatoxins exhibit a yellow-green one.

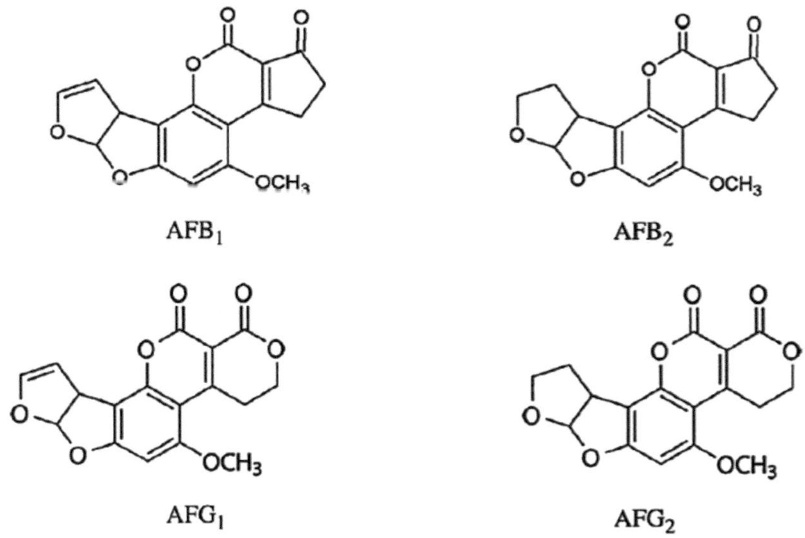

Figure 1.
Aflatoxins molecular structures.

Aspergillus species are very diverse and can adapt to a wide range of environmental conditions [4] but mainly they are found in hot humid climates typically in tropical and subtropical regions, most significantly, between 40°S and 40°N latitude [5]. *Aspergillus* sp. optimal growth happens at a temperature of 25°C with a minimum water activity of 0.75, however, their secondary metabolites production starts at 10–12°C with the most toxic metabolites produced at 25°C with 0.95 water activity [1]. Those growth patterns differ between different strains of *Aspergillus* sp., for example, optimal growth temperature of the most significant strains, *A. flavus* and *A. parasiticus*, occurs at 33°C and 35°C, respectively [6, 7].

On-field, normally, *A. flavus*, that naturally colonize the aerial parts of the plant including leaves and flowers, produces B aflatoxins while *A. parasiticus*, which are usually found in the soil environment, produce B and G aflatoxins. As for aflatoxin M_1 and M_2 they are produced *in vivo* as the hydroxylated metabolites of aflatoxins B_1 and B_2, respectively. Naturally, the colonization rate of *Aspergillus sp.* and the degree of contamination with AFs are determined by several factors including; temperature, a_w, and humidity. Additionally, contamination is promoted due to stress or physical damage to the crop especially due to drought episodes, insect infestation, rain showers during pre-harvest, poor harvest timing, and insufficient drying before storage [1]. *Aspergillus* species can further colonize the crop during storage, specifically under uncontrolled conditions that allow their domination such as increased humidity and temperature. Many types of crops and plants that are used as a source of human food or animal feed are prone to colonization by *Aspergillus* sp. and subsequent contamination with AFs, such as wheat, barley, maize, rice, sorghum, soy, peanuts, nuts, oilseeds, legumes, spices, herbs, etc. [1, 2, 8–10].

1.1.1 Aflatoxin B1 (AFB1)

Among all identified aflatoxins, AFB1 is considered the most common and it accounts for almost 75% of worldwide AF contamination in food and feed [3].

AFB1 production is the result of a complex biosynthetic pathway that involves at least 27 enzymatic reactions [11]. The genes responsible for enzymatic coding are grouped in a cluster and their expression depends on two cluster-specific regulators: *aflR* and *aflS* [11]. Additional genes are also involved in the pathway including *aflD* [11]. AFB1 is the most potent carcinogen among all mycotoxins [12, 13]. It is also the most hepatotoxic and hepatocarcinogenic agent, therefore, it poses the highest concern for food safety and health. Worldwide, AFB1 have been the main aflatoxin causing most cases of aflatoxicoses. According to Paulin et al., AFB1 can cause "acute toxicity, chronic toxicity, carcinogenicity, teratogenicity, genotoxicity, and immunotoxicity" [1]. Many epidemiological studies have demonstrated AFB1 as the major contributor to hepatocarcinoma cases [14] and it had been estimated that 4.2–28.2% of HCC cases worldwide are caused by AFB1 [15]. And due to its well-documented carcinogenicity, the IARC classified AFB1 as carcinogenic to humans (group 1) [16].

Upon intake of contaminated food, AFB1 gets rapidly absorbed through a passive mechanism in the gastrointestinal tract. It is then metabolized in the liver where it gets converted by cytochrome P-450 into aflatoxin-8, 9-epoxide, hydroxylated into a less potent form AFM1, and demethylated into aflatoxin P_1 that is excreted in the urine [12, 14]. The resulting epoxide is highly reactive so it binds to DNA or protein molecules. Binding to a protein molecule in the liver eventually causes hepatotoxicity while binding to a DNA molecule affects the genetic code through transversion of a guanine (G) molecule to thymine (T), therefore, mutating the P53 gene that codes for tumor suppression hence allowing the formation of tumors and leading eventually to hepatocellular carcinoma (HCC) (**Figure 2**) [12, 14, 17].

1.1.2 Aflatoxin M1 (AFM1)

AFM1 is the hydroxylated metabolite of AFB1 formed in the liver (**Figures 2** and **3**). Once produced, it gets absorbed by the mammary glands and secreted in the milk of mammals. AFM1, therefore, contaminates milk and dairy products such as cheese and yogurt due to its capacity to stay intact during milk pasteurization, treatment, and fermentation [18]. AFM1 is less toxic than AFB1 and possess 2–10% of its carcinogenic potency [19]. Nevertheless, AFM1 is capable of binding to DNA leading eventually to hepatocellular carcinoma. The findings of many studies that discussed the carcinogenicity of AFM1 led to its reclassification as carcinogenic to human (group 1) by the IARC in 2002 after it was for long classified as possibly carcinogenic to humans (group 2B) [16]. AFM1 presents a particular risk for infants and children due to the vulnerability of their immune systems, their low body weights, and their high consumption of milk.

1.2 Health effects of AFs

Aflatoxins' presence is recognized as a global food safety concern by the World Health Organization since they exhibit several toxic effects on animals and humans. The diseases caused by exposure to aflatoxins are referred to as "aflatoxicosis" that could be acute or chronic. The toxic effects exhibited by AFs depend on several factors such as age, gender, intake dosage, exposure duration, and nutritional status. Acute aflatoxicosis is prevalent when individuals are exposed to food contaminated with high doses of AFs and its symptoms include abdominal pain, vomiting, diarrhea, pulmonary edema, cerebral edema, anorexia, fatty liver, jaundice, depression, and photosensitivity [20]. Acute poisoning is more prevalent in developing countries due

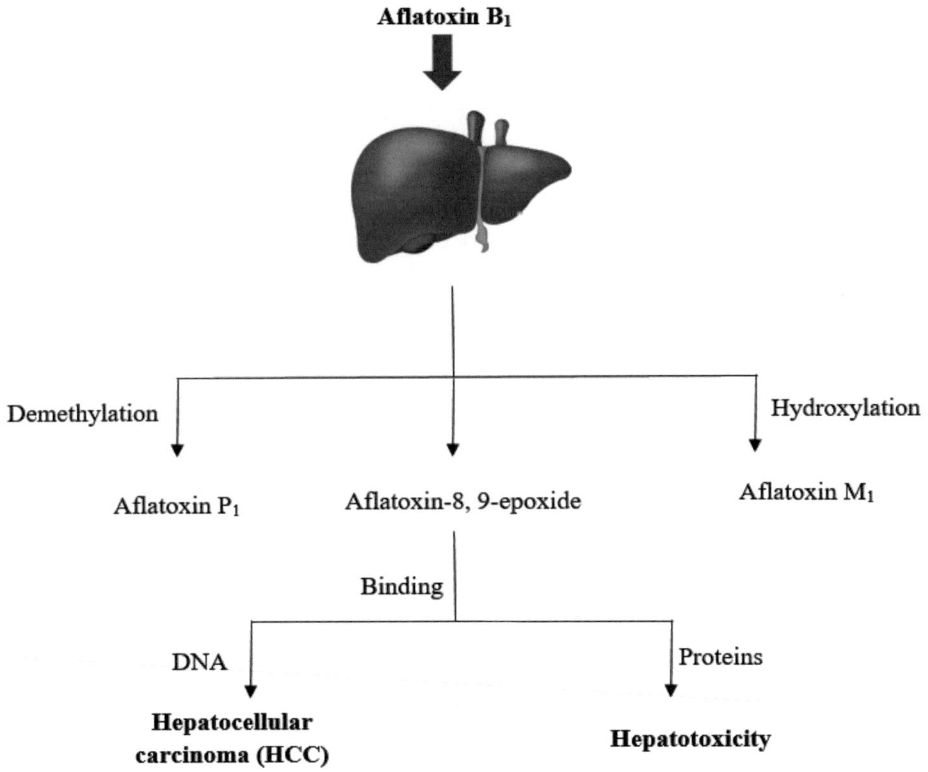

Figure 2.
AFB1 metabolism.

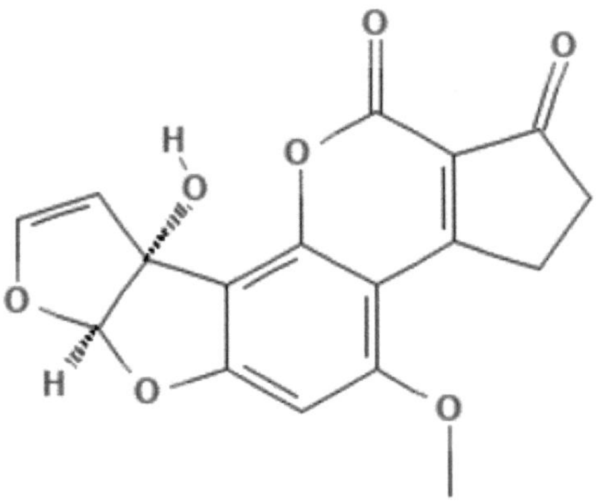

Figure 3.
AFM1 chemical structure.

to the increased risk of contamination of staple food, lack of food security, absence of AF awareness, and lack of regulatory limits. For example, in Eastern Kenia in 2004, acute liver failure was diagnosed in 317 individuals of which 125 people died later due to acute aflatoxicosis caused by consuming contaminated home-grown maize [21]. Acute aflatoxicosis presents a risk to animals, as well, due to their exposure to AFs through contaminated feed, and the susceptibility varies among different species. Acute aflatoxicosis in animals lead to several complications including decreased weight gain, reduction in egg or milk production, decreased feed conversion, and increased vulnerability to infectious diseases [20].

Chronic aflatoxicosis, on the other hand, is caused by being exposed to low doses of AFs for an extended period and results in immune suppression and cancer. The liver is the primary target organ for AFs and chronic consumption could lead to liver cancer, especially when coupled with hepatitis B and/or C virus since those viruses interact synergistically with AF causing an increased risk of hepatocellular carcinoma (HCC) [21]. Many toxicological studies demonstrated the carcinogenicity of AFs in many species including mice, rats, hamsters, monkeys, and ducks. AFs have been demonstrated as mutagenic compounds that can alter DNA leading to changes in chromosomes and mutations in genetic codes [22]. Enough evidence, therefore, lead to the classification of AFs as "group 1 carcinogen to humans" by the IARC [16]. AFs can also lead to other liver diseases such as cirrhosis and hepatomegaly [21]. Additionally, chronic exposure to AFs have been shown to affect immunity through decreased antibody production, reduced cell-mediated immunity, and decreased resistance to fungal, bacterial, and parasitic secondary infection [20, 21]. AFs exposure may also lead to low birth weights since exposure can occur in the uterus through a trans-placental pathway. Impaired child growth can be also caused by being exposed to AFs, especially since exposure is higher in children due to their low body weights which leads to more toxic effects. For example, a follow-up study in Benin showed that there was a strong negative correlation between aflatoxin-albumin adducts and height increase in children over 8 months period [23, 24]. Similarly, in the Gambia, a follow-up study demonstrated a strong effect of AF exposure during pregnancy on the infant's growth rate during their first year of life [24, 25].

2. The Mediterranean region

2.1 Region and climate

The Mediterranean is an intercontinental sea located between Europe, North Africa, and Western Asia [26]. Its surface area covers around 2.5 million km^2 and is surrounded by a total of 22 countries including Lebanon, Cyprus, Egypt, Morocco, Spain, Italy, France, etc. [27, 28].

The Mediterranean climate is characterized by mild wet winters and warm dry sunny summers with temperature and humidity variations among different countries [28]. The sea itself is surrounded by vast land areas and acts as a heat reservoir and a source of moisture for them [28]. The climate in the North and South Mediterranean differs mainly due to the fact that the former includes countries with a west coastal climate (e.g. Spain, Turkey, Cyprus) while the latter includes countries with a subtropical desert climate (e.g. Morocco, Syria) [28, 29]. The summer duration range from 2 to 7 months starting from North to South region.

2.2 Agricultural sector

Agriculture in the Mediterranean countries plays a crucial role in the economy as it provides a main source of income and employment, and ensures food security in the region. Around 28% of the Mediterranean land is devoted to agriculture with discrepancies between different countries depending on economic development, industrialization, urbanization, etc. [30].

Agriculture in the Mediterranean basin depends on irrigation, especially in the long hot dry summer seasons. Precipitation across the region is also subject to high inter-annual and seasonal variations, therefore, making it essential for farmers to provide irrigation to maintain crop diversification and assure high quality and yields of crops. Generally, around 21% of cultivated agricultural lands in the area are irrigated, with the main irrigation system being surface irrigation despite its low efficiency.

The Mediterranean region has some unique environmental characteristics that shape its agricultural production. First, its seasonal variation is characterized by rainy mild winters and long hot dry summers. Second, its terrain, in which the presence of coastal plains that support summer agriculture are backed up by low hills or mountains that help provide at sometimes snow water for irrigation in the summer.

Climate patterns also affect agricultural products along the Mediterranean Basin, for example, temperate crops can be cultivated in rainy seasons, while sub-tropical crops can be grown in summer seasons. Several agricultural commodities are produced in the Mediterranean region, first, traditional permanent crops like olives, grapes, fruits, vegetables, and dates. Most of the grapes grown in the Mediterranean region are used for wine production, additionally, grapes are also cultivated for table grapes, currants, and sultanas. Similarly, olives are used to produce olive oil and which amounts to 99% of the world's output with the main producers being Italy, Spain, and Greece [30]. As for fruits and vegetables, the Mediterranean basin production accounts for approximately 16% and 13% of the world's fruits and vegetable production, respectively. The Mediterranean region also accounts for 85% of world hazelnut output, 36% of dates, 55% of pulses, etc. [30].

Second, cereals are produced in the region specifically wheat, maize, barley, and rice which contribute to 90% of cereal production [31]. While most of the Mediterranean countries produce cereals, their yields are not enough for local consumption, therefore, most of the countries depend on imports and store cereals for long durations to ensure an adequate and continuous supply. On an overall scale, 16% of total world wheat output is produced in the Mediterranean, with France being the main producer and the only exporter country followed by Turkey, Spain, Italy, and Egypt [30].

2.3 Aflatoxins in the Mediterranean

The climate of the Mediterranean is in general inductive to fungal attacks and mycotoxin production, in addition to other factors, such as prevalence of pests, irrigation systems, droughts, agricultural practices, storage techniques, etc. Generally, the most important mycotoxins in the Mediterranean basin are aflatoxins, ochratoxin A, trichothecenes, and fumonisins with variations in the type and level of each mycotoxin in each country and in different regions [32]. Aflatoxin contamination specifically of dried fruits is most frequent in the southern and eastern parts of the basin including African and Asian countries [32]. Crops such as peanuts, pistachios, and maize are also reported to be contaminated with aflatoxins in the Mediterranean basin [32].

AFM1 is also frequent in Mediterranean countries and has been reported in many studies among different countries due to the presence of AFB1 in the feed either due to field contamination or improper storage practices.

2.4 Aflatoxins regulations in Mediterranean countries

Previous studies done in the Mediterranean region have showed a frequency of aflatoxins contamination specifically AFB1 and AFM1. As a control measure,

DOI: http://dx.doi.org/10.5772/intechopen.108534

Country	Commodity	AFT (μg/kg)	AFB1 (μg/kg)	AFM1 (μg/l)
Algeria	Cereals	—	10	—
Cyprus	Cereals, pulses, oilseeds, dried fruits, sesame, and their food products	5	—	—
Egypt	Peanuts, oilseeds, cereals, and their products	10	5	—
European Union	All cereals and all products derived from cereals	4	2	—
	Maize and rice to be subjected to sorting or other physical treatment before human consumption	10	5	—
	Groundnuts (peanuts) and other oilseeds and processed products intended for direct human consumption or use as an ingredient in foodstuff	4	2	—
	Almonds and pistachios for direct human consumption or use as an ingredient in foodstuff	10	8	—
	Hazelnuts and Brazil nuts for direct human consumption or use as an ingredient in foodstuff	10	5	—
	Other tree nuts for direct human consumption or use as an ingredient in foodstuff	4	2	—
	Spices	10	5	
	Raw milk, heat-treated milk and milk for the manufacture of milk-based products	—	—	0.05
	Infant formula	—	—	0.025

Country	Commodity	AFT (μg/kg)	AFB1 (μg/kg)	AFM1 (μg/l)
France	Peanuts, pistachios, almonds, and oilseeds	—	1	—
	All cereals	—	5	—
	White wheat flour	—	3	—
	Raw wheat bran	—	10	—
	Whole wheat flour	—	5	—
	All vegetable oils	—	5	—
	Children food products	—	1	—
	Milk	—	—	0.05
	Milk powder	—	—	0.5
	Liquid milk for infants	—	—	0.03
	Milk powder for infants	—	—	0.3
Greece	Dried fruits, peanuts, hazelnuts, walnuts, pistachios, almond, pumpkin seeds, sunflower seeds, pine seeds, apricot seeds, maize,	—	5	—
Italy	All foods	10	5	—
	Spices	40	20	—
Lebanon	Cereals	4	2	—
	Milk	—	—	0.05
Morocco	Cereals and cereal-based products	4	2	—
	Milk	—	—	0.05
Spain	All food for human consumption	10	5	—
Syria	Fluid milk	—	—	0.2
	Powdered milk	—	—	0.05
Tunisia	Cereals	—	2	—

Country	Commodity	AFT (µg/kg)	AFB1 (µg/kg)	AFM1 (µg/l)
Turkey	All foods	20	5	—
	Infant foods	2	—	—
	Milk and milk products	—	—	0.5

Table 1.
AFT, AFB1, and AFM1 maximum tolerable limits in some Mediterranean countries [33–36].

Mediterranean countries have adopted different regulations while specifically many European countries follow the European Commission legislation (**Table 1**).

3. Climate change patterns' effects on aflatoxins

3.1 Preharvest effects

Environmental conditions are the main driving factors of fungal attack patterns and mycotoxin contamination in foodstuff, therefore, emerging climatic conditions may induce changes in the dynamics of fungal colonization and mycotoxin production. Since the industrial revolution, production patterns and human activities including agricultural production, food processing, fossil fuel combustion, and others have been contributing to increased pollution and greenhouse gases emission. The increased accumulation of those gases in the atmosphere is the main driving factor of global warming and climate change.

With the change in climatic conditions, global warming is expected to induce an increase in global temperatures that are expected to rise by 1.5–4.5°C by the end of the twenty-first century [37], along with an increased accumulation of carbon dioxide in the atmosphere, increase in precipitation, the dominance of extreme weather conditions such as heat and cold waves, and an increase in the incidence of flooding and droughts [38].

Climate change patterns will have a direct effect on agriculture characterized by a decrease in plant resilience and yields, deterioration of crop quality, and an increase in pest and insect population, spread, and attacks [39]. Additionally, changes in global temperatures can lead to early maturing and ripening of crops in certain areas that will lead to a change in the patterns of harvest, drying, and storage.

All those factors, will in turn affect food security since a change in fungal attack and mycotoxin production properties are expected [40]. Hence, according to the European Food Safety Authority, some geographical regions will have advantageous effects while others will experience detrimental ones according to the forecasted environmental changes [41]. The Mediterranean region, specifically, was reported to be highly affected by the ongoing climate change as it was reported to be warming 20% faster than the global average by the "Mediterranean Action Plan Barcelona Convention" of the UN environment program creating a hotspot region of climate change. In addition to that, changes affecting the Mediterranean region include the increase in the frequency and intensity of droughts, the decrease in precipitation in the eastern Mediterranean coupled by an increase in temperature of 2–3°C [42]. The number of hot days characterized by temperatures above 30°C is also likely to increase in a number of countries including Spain, Morocco, Algeria, the center of Italy, the Balkans, and central Turkey [30].

As reported by Medina et al., Southern Europe and the Mediterranean basin will undergo significant changes that will eventually cause an increase in fungal colonization and mycotoxin frequency [43]. This change affects *Aspergillus species* colonization and aflatoxins production as warm conditions favor the attack and growth of their producers, leading to their frequency in regions once considered as temperate and different from their typical production areas in tropical and sub-tropical regions [44].

Additionally, climate change will reproduce suitable and favorable environmental conditions of droughts, high temperatures, and humidity for *Aspergillus* colonization and aflatoxins and their precursors' production. Indeed, droughts are considered an important trigger for biosynthesis of aflatoxins and according to Valencia-Quintana et al. the sudden change in precipitation and drought patterns followed by increased humidity, temperature, and CO_2 levels will directly affect the expression of the regulatory and structural genes (*aflR* and *aflD*) implicated in aflatoxins biosynthesis [44]. The Mediterranean region already has marked summer droughts, prolonged heat waves, regular flooding, and varied precipitation volume [30]. However, those climatic patterns are all liable to intensify as according to the forecasts for the mid-twenty-first century, extreme drought situations will become more prevalent and the number of dry days is expected to increase by at least three weeks every year specifically on the northern shores of the western Mediterranean, in countries such as Portugal, Spain, France, Italy, Croatia, Montenegro, and Turkey which can increase the frequency of *Asperillius* sp. and aflatoxin contamination [30].

On the other hand, elevated CO_2 atmospheric levels can further lead to aflatoxin contamination, specifically, as reported by many studies, cause the environment where the crops are cultivated is expected to markedly change due to the elevated concentrations of CO_2 that are projected to double or triple from a concentration of 350 ppm to a range of 700–1000 ppm [45]. According to Medina et al., AFB1 production was stimulated under climate change scenarios related to elevated CO_2 levels, especially when coupled with drought stress [45]. The same study, showed no effect on the growth of *Aspergillus* sp. in case of increased CO_2 levels, while the relative increase was reported in the structural *aflD* and the regulatory *aflR* genes, suggesting a significant impact on the biosynthetic pathway involved in aflatoxins production, particularly at an elevated temperature of 37°C and under water stress conditions [45]. In what relates to the Mediterranean region, the annual greenhouse gas emissions account for around 5.4 tonnes per capita, compared to 4 tonnes per capita as a global average [30]. Additionally, the northern part of the region is responsible for 70% of total Mediterranean CO_2 emissions which is approximate 8% of the world's total emissions [30]. Certain countries are also expected to witness a blast in greenhouse gas emissions including Lebanon, Turkey, Algeria, Malta, and Tunisia [30]. Therefore, extra CO_2 accumulation will result in the region and will affect fungal attack patterns in a way favoring *Aspegillus* sp. infections and the production of aflatoxins.

Finally, several studies suggest that global warming is causing pests and diseases to move towards the poles, which may lead to damage of staple crops and the decreased resilience of plants, making them more prone to infection with *Aspergillus* sp. and contamination with aflatoxins [38, 46].

3.2 Harvest and postharvest effects

The changed climatic conditions can lead to early maturing of the plant and can create favorable conditions for *Aspergillus* sp. infestation and aflatoxin production at time of harvest, especially upon the dominance of high temperatures and humidity. Following harvest, drying is considered an important stage in aflatoxin control, so upon reaching adequate water activity levels, crops can be admitted safely into storage. However, with the dominance of extreme environmental conditions, especially, high humidity, reaching adequate water activity before storage would be hard to achieve. Additionally, the sudden patterns of rainfall, precipitation, and dew can lead to the soaking of crops and the failure of the drying procedure specifically if sun-drying was performed in the open fields [47].

The challenge, therefore, is preserving the crop from *Aspergillus* sp. at the time of storage since in case it was present, most likely it would keep on growing and metabolizing aflatoxins [48]. According to Magan et al., stored crops are usually alive respiring media during postharvest in storage facilities, therefore, it is extremely important to consider the interacting abiotic and biotic factors in assessing the changes related to climate change [47] Notably, it is essential to control temperature and relative humidity during storage and maintain them at levels below 10°C and 70%, respectively, which would be challenging in traditional storage facilities prevalent in some Mediterranean countries in climate change scenarios [49]. Therefore, under uncontrolled storage conditions, such as in the presence of pests that are facilitated by increased attack patterns due to climate change scenarios, and upon the increased growth and multiplication of different bacterial and fungal species in the presence of elevated temperatures and humidity, increased water evaporation and condensation could result, leading to damp conditions that support *Aspergillus* sp. metabolism and growth, subsequent aflatoxin production, and the formation of internal pockets of contamination [49]. Therefore, with climate change scenarios, aflatoxin contamination is expected to increase in the Mediterranean basin during storage, specifically since countries of the region rely heavily on imports and storage of grains. This might lead to increased AFB1 in food and feed and subsequent AFM1 contamination of milk and dairy products.

3.3 Recent occurrence data of aflatoxins in the Mediterranean region under changing climate scenarios

Until recent years, aflatoxin contamination was not a food safety concern in the Mediterranean region, specifically in the European part, however, the change in climate patterns has altered this situation and created an increased risk of *Aspergillus* sp. attacks and aflatoxin contamination in regions once considered as temperate [50].

Many studies are indicating that aflatoxins are increasingly detected in parts of the Mediterranean, specifically, southern Europe, in quantities not observed before. In Italy, in 2003 and 2004, a set of dry and hot episodes led to the colonization of *A. flavus* and subsequent aflatoxin production in maize intended for animal feed [44, 51]. In Serbia, during the year 2012, and due to hot and dry weather, 69% of maize samples were contaminated with aflatoxins [38]. In Hungary as well, a reported increase in aflatoxin contamination was attributed to climate change conditions in 2012 [38]. In the summer season of the same year and due to elevated temperatures and drought conditions, a shift in fungal attack patterns was observed in Northern Italy, where a switch from *Fusarium* sp. to *A. flavus* was observed in maize that resulted in subsequent production of AFM1 in the dairy chain [45]. Similarly, an outbreak of aflatoxin contamination of maize was reported in the Balkan region in 2013 [37].

In 2015, several noncompliances with the limits specified by the European Commission were also reported in North Italy [37]. Additionally, in the last years, the dominance of hot and dry seasons led to *A. flavus* infections in maize in several Mediterranean countries including Romania and Spain [52]. *A. flavus* infection was also observed in gape vineyards in Lebanon due to increased temperatures where usually *A. carbonarius* that generally produce ochratoxin A are traditionally detected [53].

According to Battilani et al., that investigated the probability of emergence of AFB1 in European cereals due to climate change, there will be a clear increase in the risk of aflatoxin contamination in countries such as Spain, Italy, Greece, Portugal, Bulgaria, Cyprus, ad Turkey [41].

The increased risk of AFB1 contamination is most likely to appear as well as AFM1 contamination in milk and dairy products. Several previous studies as well have reported AFM1 contamination in a number of Mediterranean countries. For example, AFM1 contamination was reported in countries such as Spain, Turkey, Lebanon, Egypt, and Syria where AFM1 was found in 33%, 12%, 59%, 38%, and 14% of raw milk samples, respectively [54, 55]. Also, AFM1 levels in raw milk samples from Bosnia and Herzegovina and Croatia were reported at 6.22 ng/kg and 5.65 ng/kg, respectively [56]. Additionally, AFM1 contamination was reported in dairy products from the region; in Lebanon, Portugal, Italy, and Turkey AFM1 was reported in 66%, 4%, 80%, and 40% of different dairy products, respectively [55–57]. The contamination with AFM1 can be directly attributed to AFB1 presence in animal feed that might be due to on-field or during storage contamination.

4. Aflatoxins economic impact and control

4.1 Impact on global food chain and economy

Mycotoxins prevalence presents a global issue and contamination of crops takes place worldwide impacting the economy significantly. The Food and Agriculture Organization of the United Nations estimated that "approximately 25% of cereals produced around the world are contaminated with mycotoxins". However, recently, Eskola et al. reported that this figure underestimates worldwide occurrence and considered that 60–80% of crops are contaminated above detectable levels [58]. Eskola et al. attributed this increase to improvements in analytical methods' sensitivity in addition to the possible impact of climate change [58]. In the United States of America, for example, mycotoxins result in crop losses that average 932 million dollars per year and worldwide annual losses due to those natural toxins amount to around 1 billion metric tons of food and food products as estimated by the Food and Agriculture Organization (FAO). More specifically, losses due to aflatoxin contamination in maize top up to 160 million dollars annually in the U.S.A. [50]. Developing regions, such as Africa where losses are alarming, might be affected seriously by aflatoxin contamination problems due to several aspects including; export rejections, a subsequent decrease in the market value of contaminated products, and decrease in crops marketability. This effect was evident since according to Gbashi et al., losses in sub-Saharan Africa amount to a total of 450 million dollars representing 38% of global losses in agricultural commodities due to aflatoxins [50, 59]. The presence of aflatoxins may disrupt the world trade system, as well, since many basic foodstuffs such as vegetables, fruits, dried fruits, nuts, oilseeds, cocoa beans, coffee beans, herbs, spices, milk, dairy products, beer, and animal feed can be contaminated. And ideally, to get rid of aflatoxins, contaminated commodities should be destroyed resulting, therefore, in huge losses. Alternatively, in some cases contaminated crops are redirected to be used as animal feed, the thing that may cause undesirable consequences including reduced growth rates, illness in animals, and the carry-over of residues or byproducts of aflatoxins into animal products such as milk and dairy products that further augment the economic problem of mycotoxins. In addition to that, aflatoxins impact economy due to the cost of analysis and strategies in order to control it, and to the burden it could add to healthcare cost due to health problems it induce.

4.2 Aflatoxin control across the food chain

Aflatoxin production is generally unavoidable when the environmental conditions are permissible, however, some control strategies can be applied from the first stages of the food chain until the last stages which may decrease contamination of the final product (**Figure 4**) [39].

Starting from preharvest stage good agricultural practices can be applied including tiling, deep plowing, crop rotation, proper irrigation methods, weed removal, timing the production cycle, and use of high-quality seeds and disease-resistant cultivars, etc. [60–62] Following that, proper harvest is crucial to decrease the chances of contamination. Strategies at harvest include performing harvest in a dry weather and at a fast rate, checking for signs of fungal contamination and separating diseased crops from intact ones, and properly use clean equipment to avoid mechanical damage to crops [60]. Following that, drying should be performed in controlled conditions of temperature and humidity, and it is very crucial to reach the desired safe moisture content before storage [60].

Storage is a very critical stage for aflatoxin control. During that phase, controlled conditions of temperature and humidity should be applied to prevent fungal growth and subsequent mycotoxin production. *Aspergillus* sp. can become of important significance in case storage was done in classic silos and containers under uncontrolled conditions. According to Villers 2014, "Aflatoxin-producing molds grow exponentially in conventional multi-month storage as a result of a combination of heat and high humidity" leading, therefore, to increased aflatoxin contamination in storage [63]. Additionally, classic storage facilities are not well sealed and insulated against outer environmental factors, so this would lead to water evaporation due to grain metabolism followed by condensation which will eventually increase water activity of the crop and lead to the development of internal pockets of fungal contamination including *Aspergilluss* sp. That will lead to subsequent aflatoxins production and increased contamination [49]. Therefore, it is very important to control temperature and relative humidity and maintain them at levels below 10°C and 70%, respectively through the whole period of storage [39]. It is also essential to weatherproof and seal storage facilities against weather conditions and pest attacks.

Across the food chain, several decontamination methods could be applied, either biological, physical, or chemical to decrease aflatoxin contamination, however, up till now there is no technique developed that has proved to be simultaneously effective

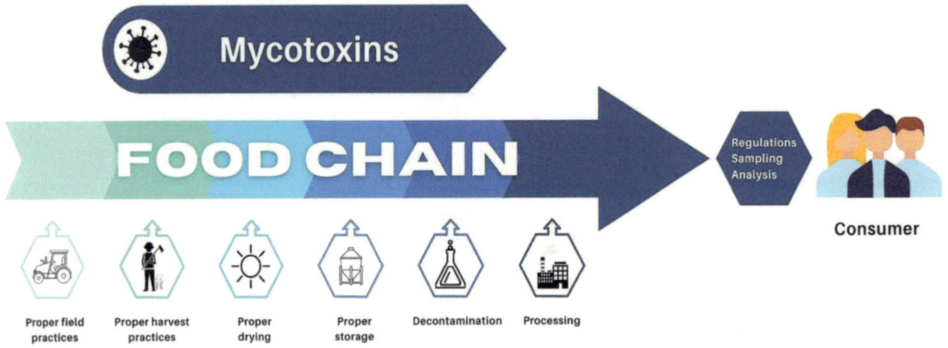

Figure 4.
Strategies to decrease aflatoxin contamination through the whole food chain [49].

and practical at the industrial scale [39]. Recently, increased concentration has been applied on the development of novel techniques that can be used to naturally bind aflatoxins in food. Examples of such developments include the usage of lactic acid bacteria [64] and their biofilms [65] to bind AFM1 in milk. In addition, other adsorbents such as chitin and shrimp shells were also highly effective in AFM1 removal from liquids [66]. As for processing, the highly stable nature of aflatoxins renders them highly resistant to any processing techniques including the application of heat in procedures like pasteurization.

Finally, and before admission to consumers, to ensure the safety of their population health, many countries around the world have set regulations for aflatoxin in food in the forms of maximum tolerable limits (MTL). These limits are established based on the fact that it is practically hard to achieve zero contamination in many foodstuff and those are decided according to the tolerable daily exposure to aflatoxins at levels that do not pose health risks.

5. Conclusion

Climate change patterns are expected to induce changes creating more favorable conditions for *Aspergillus* sp. attacks, growth, and metabolism. Subsequently, aflatoxins production is expected to increase specifically AFB1. The Mediterranean region, once considered as a temperate region, is considered to be highly affected by the ongoing changes, therefore, contamination with AFB1 in several commodities is expected in addition to the contamination of AFM1 in the milk and dairy products chain which presents emerging threats on food safety, security, and trade.

Finally, more research is needed to determine emerging toxin production patterns, agricultural mitigation practices, and strategies to reduce the impact of contamination on consumers' health. Additionally, studies particularly designed to explore the fungal attack patterns and mycotoxin production tailored to the Mediterranean region are required.

Author details

Rouaa Daou, Jean Claude Assaf* and André El Khoury
Faculty of Sciences, Centre d'Analyses et de Recherche (CAR), Unité de Recherche Technologies et Valorisation agro-Alimentaire (UR-TVA), Saint-Joseph University of Beirut, Mar Roukos, Lebanon

*Address all correspondence to: jeanclaude.assaf@net.usj.edu.lb

References

[1] Lizárraga-Paulín EG. In: Moreno-Martínez E, editor. Aflatoxins and their Impact on Human and Animal Health: An Emerging Problem. Rijeka, London, UK: IntechOpen; 2011. p. Ch. 13. DOI: 10.5772/26196

[2] Bennett JW, Klich M. Mycotoxins. Clinical Microbiology Reviews. 2003;**16**(3):497-516

[3] Wacoo AP, Wendiro D, Vuzi PC, Hawumba JF. Methods for detection of aflatoxins in agricultural food crops. Journal of Applied Chemistry. 2014;**2014**:1-15

[4] Paulussen C, Hallsworth JE, Álvarez-Pérez S, Nierman WC, Hamill PG, Blain D, et al. Ecology of aspergillosis: Insights into the pathogenic potency of Aspergillus fumigatus and some other Aspergillus species. Microbial Biotechnology. 2017;**10**(2):296-322

[5] Acur A, Arias RS, Odongo S, Tuhaise S, Ssekandi J, Adriko J, et al. Genetic diversity of aflatoxin-producing Aspergillus flavus isolated from selected groundnut growing agro-ecological zones of Uganda. BMC Microbiology. 2020;**20**(1):252. Available from: https://pubmed.ncbi.nlm.nih.gov/32795262

[6] Schmidt-Heydt M, Rüfer CE, Abdel-Hadi A, Magan N, Geisen R. The production of aflatoxin B1 or G 1 by Aspergillus parasiticus at various combinations of temperature and water activity is related to the ratio of aflS to aflR expression. Mycotoxin Research. 2010;**26**(4):241-246

[7] Bailly S, El Mahgubi A, Carvajal-Campos A, Lorber S, Puel O, Oswald IP, et al. Occurrence and identification of Aspergillus section flavi in the context of the emergence of aflatoxins in French Maize. Toxins (Basel). 2018;**10**(12):525. Available from: https://pubmed.ncbi.nlm.nih.gov/30544593

[8] Marchese S, Polo A, Ariano A, Velotto S, Costantini S, Severino L. Aflatoxin B1 and M1: Biological properties and their involvement in cancer development. Toxins (Basel). May 2018;**10**(6):1-19

[9] Assaf JC, Nahle S, Louka N, Chokr A, Atoui A, El Khoury A. Assorted methods for decontamination of Aflatoxin. Toxins (Basel). 2020;**11**(304):1-23

[10] Daou R, Joubrane K, Khabbaz LR, Maroun RG, Ismail A, El Khoury A. Aflatoxin B1 and ochratoxin A in imported and Lebanese wheat and -products. Food Additives & Contaminants: Part B. 2021;**14**(3):1-9. DOI: 10.1080/19393210.2021.1933203

[11] Caceres I, Khoury AA, Khoury RE, Lorber S, Oswald IP, Khoury AE, et al. Aflatoxin biosynthesis and genetic regulation: A review. Toxins (Basel). Feb 2020;**12**(3):1-28

[12] Ahmed Adam MA, Tabana YM, Musa KB, Sandai DA. Effects of different mycotoxins on humans, cell genome and their involvement in cancer (review). Oncology Reports. 2017;**37**(3):1321-1336

[13] Bullerman L, Bianchini A. Stability of mycotoxins during food processing. International Journal of Food Microbiology. 2007;**119**:140-146

[14] Hamid AS, Tesfamariam IG, Zhang Y, Zhang ZG. Aflatoxin B1-induced hepatocellular carcinoma in developing countries: Geographical distribution, mechanism of action

and prevention. Oncology Letters. 2013;**5**(4):1087-1092

[15] Küçükçakan B, Hayrulai-Musliu Z. Challenging role of dietary Aflatoxin B1 exposure and hepatitis B infection on risk of hepatocellular carcinoma. Open Access Macedonian Journal of Medical Sciences. 2015;**3**:363

[16] International Agency for Research on Cancer. International Agency for Research on Cancer Iarc Monographs on the Evaluation of Carcinogenic Risks To Humans. Iarc Monogr Eval Carcinog Risks To Humans [Internet]. Vol. 80. 2002. pp. 27, 338. Available from: http://scholar.google.com/scholar?hl=en&btnG=Search&q=intitle:INTERNATIONAL+AGENCY+FOR+RESEARCH+ON+CANCER+IARC+MONOGRAPHS+ON+THE+EVALUATION+OF+CARCINOGENIC+RISKS+TO+HUMANS#2%5Cnhttp://scholar.google.com/scholar?hl=en&btnG=Search&q=intitle:International+Ag

[17] Williams JH, Phillips TD, Jolly PE, Stiles JK, Jolly CM, Aggarwal D. Human aflatoxicosis in developing countries: A review of toxicology, exposure, potential health consequences, and interventions. The American Journal of Clinical Nutrition. 2004;**80**(5):1106-1122

[18] Flores-Flores ME, Lizarraga E, López de Cerain A, González-Peñas E. Presence of mycotoxins in animal milk: A review. Food Control. 2015;**53**:163-176

[19] Schrenk D, Bignami M, Bodin L, Chipman JK, del Mazo J, Grasl-Kraupp B, et al. Risk assessment of aflatoxins in food. EFSA Journal. 2020;**18**(3):1-112

[20] Marin S, Ramos AJ, Sanchis V. Mycotoxins: Occurrence, toxicology, and exposure assessment. Food and Chemical Toxicology. 2013;**60**:218-237. DOI: 10.1016/j.fct.2013.07.047

[21] Gong YY, Watson S, Routledge M. Aflatoxin exposure and associated human health effects, a review of epidemiological studies. Food Safety. 2016;**4**:14-27

[22] Sarma UP, Bhetaria PJ, Devi P, Varma A. Aflatoxins: Implications on health. Indian Journal of Clinical Biochemistry. 2017;**32**(2):124-133

[23] Gong YY, Hounsa A, Egal S, Turner P, Sutcliffe A, Hall A, et al. Postweaning exposure to aflatoxin results in impaired child growth: A longitudinal study in Benin, West Africa. Environmental Health Perspectives. 2004;**112**:1334-1338

[24] Kensler T, Roebuck B, Wogan G, Groopman J. Aflatoxin: A 50-year odyssey of mechanistic and translational toxicology. Toxicological Sciences. 2010;**120**(Suppl):S28-S48

[25] Turner PC, Collinson AC, Cheung YB, Gong Y, Hall AJ, Prentice AM, et al. Aflatoxin exposure in utero causes growth faltering in Gambian infants. International Journal of Epidemiology. 2007;**36**(5):1119-1125

[26] De Martino L, Nazzaro F, Mancini E, De Feo V. Chapter 58—Essential oils from Mediterranean aromatic plants. In: Preedy VR, Watson RR, editors. The Mediterranean Diet. San Diego: Academic Press; 2015. pp. 649-661. Available from: https://www.sciencedirect.com/science/article/pii/B9780124078499000580

[27] Rhazi K El, Kinany K El, García-Larsen V. Socioeconomic factors for the adherence to the Mediterranean diet in North Africa: The shift from 1990 to 2019. The Mediterranean Diet. 2020:57-65

[28] Lionello P, Malanotte-Rizzoli P, Boscolo R, Alpert P, Artale V, Li L,

et al. The Mediterranean climate: An overview of the Main characteristics and issues. Developments in Earth and Environmental Sciences. 2006;**4**:1-26

[29] Katerji N, Mastrorilli M, Rana G. Water use efficiency of crops cultivated in the Mediterranean region: Review and analysis. European Journal of Agronomy. 2008;**28**(4):493-507. Available from: https://www.sciencedirect.com/science/article/pii/S1161030107001268

[30] Abdelhakim T, Antonelli A, Bencharif A, Bessaoud O, Dollé V, Giove R, et al. Mediterra 2008. The Future of Agriculture and Food in Mediterranean Countries [Internet]. 360 p. Available from: http://www.pressesdesciencespo.fr/resources/titles/27246100295730/extras/MEDITERRA_2008_anglais.pdf

[31] Cherif S, Cramer W, Giupponi C, Joel G, Lionello P, Marini K, et al. CLIMATE AND ENVIRONMENTAL CHANGE IN THE MEDITERRANEAN BASIN Current situation and risks for the future. First Mediterranean Assessment Report by MedECC (Mediterranean Experts on Climate and environmental Change). 2021

[32] Tsitsigiannis D, Dimakopoulou M, Antoniou P, Tjamos E. Biological control strategies of mycotoxigenic fungi and associated mycotoxins in Mediterranean basin crops. Phytopathologia Mediterranea. 2012;**51**(1):158-174

[33] Mazumder PM, Sasmal D. Mycotoxins—Limits and regulations. Ancient Science of Life. 2001;**20**(3):1-19

[34] Lahouar A, Jedidi I, Said S. Incidence, legislations and strategies of control of mycotoxins in North African countries. International Food Resarch Journal. 2018;**25**(6):2229-2247

[35] Bouafifssa Y, Manyes L, Rahouti M, Mañes J, Berrada H, Zinedine A, et al. Multi-occurrence of twenty mycotoxinsin pasta and a risk assessment in the Moroccan population. Toxins (Basel). 2018;**10**(11):432. Available from: https://pubmed.ncbi.nlm.nih.gov/30373176

[36] Ghanem I, Orfi M. Aflatoxin M1 in raw, pasteurized and powdered milk available in the Syrian market. Food Control. 2009;**20**(6):603-605. DOI: 10.1016/j.foodcont.2008.08.018

[37] Van Der Fels-Klerx HJ, Liu C, Battilani P. Modelling climate change impacts on mycotoxin contamination. World Mycotoxin Journal. 2016;**9**(5):717-726

[38] Medina A, Rodríguez A, Magan N. Climate change and mycotoxigenic fungi: Impacts on mycotoxin production. Current Opinion in Food Science. 2015;**5**:99-104

[39] Daou R, Joubrane K, Maroun RG, Khabbaz LR, Ismail A, El Khoury A. Mycotoxins: Factors influencing production and control strategies. AIMS Agriculture and Food. 2021;**6**(1):416-447. Available from: file:///article/id/60361b93ba35de13e07f4cb3

[40] Miraglia M, De Santis B, Brera C. Climate change: Implications for mycotoxin contamination of foods. Journal of Biotechnology. 2008;**136**:711-716

[41] Battilani P, Rossi V, Giorni P, Pietri A, Gualla A, van der Fels-Klerx HJ, et al. Modelling, predicting and mapping the emergence of aflatoxins in cereals in the EU due to climate change. EFSA Supporting Publications. 2017;**9**(1):453-454

[42] Haddad EA, Farajalla N, Camargo M, Lopes RL, Vieira FV. Climate change

in Lebanon: Higher-order regional impacts from agriculture. The Region. 2014;**1**(1):9-24

[43] Medina A, Akbar A, Baazeem A, Rodríguez A, Magan N. Climate change, food security and mycotoxins: Do we know enough? Fungal Biology Reviews. 2017;**31**(3):143-154

[44] Valencia R, Milić M, Jakšić D, Klarić M, Tenorio Arvide MG, Pérez G, et al. Environmental research and public health review environment changes, aflatoxins, and health issues, a review. International Journal of Environmental Research and Public Health. 2020;**17**:1-10

[45] Medina A, Rodriguez A, Magan N. Effect of climate change on Aspergillus flavus and aflatoxin B1 production. Frontiers in Microbiology. 2014;**5**:348

[46] Bebber D, Ramotowski M, Gurr S. Crop pests and pathogens move poleward in a warming world. Nature Climate Change. 2013;**3**(11):1-4

[47] Magan N, Medina A, Aldred D. Possible climate-change effects on mycotoxin contamination of food crops pre- and postharvest. Plant Pathology. 2011;**60**:150-163

[48] Warnatzsch EA, Reay DS, Camardo Leggieri M, Battilani P. Climate change impact on Aflatoxin contamination risk in Malawi's maize crops. Frontiers in Sustainable Food Systems. 2020;(4): 1-13. Available from: https://www.frontiersin.org/article/10.3389/fsufs.2020.591792

[49] El Khoury A, Daou R, Atoui A, Hoteit M. Mycotoxins in Lebanese Food Basket. Databse on Occurrence and Exposure. 2022; Mycotoxin Database-Lebanon.osf.io/s6rx9. Available from: https://www.researchgate.net/publication/359062063_Mycotoxin_Database-Lebanonosfios6rx9

[50] Jallow A, Xie H, Tang X, Qi Z, Li P. Worldwide aflatoxin contamination of agricultural products and foods: From occurrence to control. Comprehensive Reviews in Food Science and Food Safety. 2021;**20**(3):2332-2381. Available from: https://ift.onlinelibrary.wiley.com/doi/abs/10.1111/1541-4337.12734

[51] Giorni P, Battilani P, Magan N. Effect of solute and matric potential on in vitro growth and sporulation of strains from a new population of Aspergillus flavus isolated in Italy. Fungal Ecology. 2008;**1**:102-106

[52] Moretti A, Pascale M, Logrieco A. Mycotoxin risks under a climate change scenario in Europe. Trends in Food Science and Technology. 2018;**84**:38-40

[53] El Khoury A, Rizk T, Lteif R, Azouri H, Delia M-L, Lebrihi A. Occurrence of ochratoxin A- and aflatoxin B1-producing fungi in Lebanese grapes and ochratoxin a content in musts and finished wines during 2004. Journal of Agricultural and Food Chemistry. 2006;**54**(23):8977-8982

[54] Salari N, Kazeminia M, Vaisi-Raygani A, Jalali R, Mohammadi M. Aflatoxin M1 in Milk worldwide from 1988 to 2020: A systematic review and meta-analysis. Journal of Food Quality. 2020;**2020**:8862738. DOI: 10.1155/2020/8862738

[55] Daou R, Afif C, Joubrane K, Khabbaz LR, Maroun R, Ismail A, et al. Occurrence of aflatoxin M1 in raw, pasteurized, UHT cows' milk, and dairy products in Lebanon. Food Control. 2020;**111**(November 2019):1-7

[56] Yilmaz S, Altinci A. Incidence of aflatoxin M1 contamination in milk,

white cheese, kashar and butter from Sakarya, Turkey. Journal of Food Science and Technology. 2018;**39**(3):190-194

[57] Hassan HF, Kassaify Z. The risks associated with aflatoxins M1 occurrence in Lebanese dairy products. Food Control. 2014;**37**(1):68-72. DOI: 10.1016/j.foodcont.2013.08.022

[58] Eskola M, Kos G, Elliott CT, Hajšlová J, Mayar S, Krska R. Worldwide contamination of food-crops with mycotoxins: Validity of the widely cited "FAO estimate" of 25. Critical Reviews in Food Science and Nutrition. 2020;**60**(16):2773-2789

[59] Gbashi S, Madala NE, de Saeger S, de Boevre M, Adekoya I, Adebo OA, et al. The socio-economic impact of mycotoxin contamination in Africa. In: Njobeh PB, Stepman F, editors. Mycotoxins. Rijeka, London, UK: IntechOpen; 2019. DOI: 10.5772/intechopen.79328

[60] Golob P. On-Farm Mycotoxin Control in Food and Feed Grain. Rome: Food and Agriculture Organization of the United Nations; 2007. Available from: https://agris.fao.org/agris-search/search.do?recordID=XF2008435835

[61] Mahuku G, Sila H, Mutegi C, Kanampiu F, Narrod C, Makumbi D. Pre-harvest management is a critical practice for minimizing a flatoxin contamination of maize. Food Control. Jun 2019;**96**:219-226. DOI: 10.1016/j.foodcont.2018.08.032

[62] Rose LJ. In: Okoth S, editor. Preharvest Management Strategies and their Impact on Mycotoxigenic Fungi and Associated Mycotoxins. Rijeka, London, UK: IntechOpen; 2019. p. Ch. 3. DOI: 10.5772/intechopen.76808

[63] Villers P. Aflatoxins and safe storage. Frontiers in Microbiology. 2014;5(158):1-6. Available from: https://www.frontiersin.org/article/10.3389/fmicb.2014.00158

[64] Assaf JC, Atoui A, El Khoury A, Chokr A, Louka N. A comparative study of procedures for binding of aflatoxin M1 to lactobacillus rhamnosus GG. Brazilian Journal of Microbiology. 2017;**49**(1):120-127. Available from: https://pubmed.ncbi.nlm.nih.gov/28843807

[65] Assaf JC, El Khoury A, Chokr A, Louka N, Atoui A. A novel method for elimination of aflatoxin M1 in milk using Lactobacillus rhamnosus GG biofilm. International Journal of Dairy Technology. 2019;**72**(2):248-256. DOI: 10.1111/1471-0307.12578

[66] Assaf JC, El Khoury A, Atoui A, Louka N, Chokr A. A novel technique for aflatoxin M1 detoxification using chitin or treated shrimp shells: In vitro effect of physical and kinetic parameters on the binding stability. Applied Microbiology and Biotechnology. 2018;**102**(15):6687-6697

Chapter 2

Aflatoxin Occurrence, Detection, and Novel Strategies to Reduce Toxicity in Poultry Species

Surya Kanta Mishra and Bijaya Kumar Swain

Abstract

Aflatoxins (AF) are the commonly occurring mycotoxins produced by various *Aspergillus* species including *A. flavus, A. parasiticus*, and *A. nominus*. As secondary metabolites of these fungi, AF may contaminate a variety of food and feedstuffs, especially corn, peanuts, and cottonseed. Among the many known AFs, AFB1 is the most commonly encountered and the most toxic. In poultry, adverse effects of AF include reduction in growth rate and feed efficiency, decreased egg production and hatchability along with increased susceptibility to diseases, besides residues in food chains. Many rapid screening methods for detecting aflatoxin are available currently, namely: thin layer chromatography (TLC), HPTLC, HPLC, enzyme-linked immunosorbent assay (ELISA), monoclonal antibody kits, and affinity column chromatography, making the detection of AF precise. For field application, rapid assay kits, e.g., Aflatest of Vicam and Afla-2-cup of Romers Labs, are currently available. The most novel ways to counteract aflatoxin already accumulated in the feed could be by getting them bound to inert compounds before absorption from host's intestine. Among various classes of poultry, ducks followed by turkeys form the two most vulnerable poultry species, among others. Considering the inherently high genetic variation between duck breeds for AFB susceptibility, a genetic selection program to improve AFB resistance can be a long-term option. Further epigenetic sensitization of the AFB-susceptible poultries through mild AFB exposures is getting reported as an emerging genetic approach to counter AFB susceptibilities. The chapter discusses most of these, in greater detail.

Keywords: aflatoxin, detection method, occurrence, detoxification, poultry, susceptibility

1. Introduction

An outbreak of Turkey-X disease in the United Kingdom in 1960s following the ingestion of poultry feed containing Brazilian ground nut cake led to the discovery of a group of compounds, which are now known as aflatoxins (AFs). Chemical and microbiological investigations soon revealed that the toxic effects produced by Brazilian ground nut cake had resulted from the presence of four secondary metabolites of the mold *Aspergillus flavus* in the diet [1].

Aflatoxins (AFs) are difuranocoumarins mainly produced by two *Aspergillous* species, namely *Aspergillous flavus* and *Aspergillousparasiticus* [2]. According to their chemical structures, there are two main categories of AFs; the first category being difuranocoumaro-cyclopetene group and includes aflatoxins B1, B2 (AFB1, AFB2) while the second category is formed by the AFG1 and AFG2. The nomenclature of AFB1 and AFB2 is derived from the blue fluorescent color produced and visualized under UV light while AFG1 and AFG2 produce green fluorescent color [3, 4]. Among all the discovered mycotoxins, aflatoxins form the most elaborately researched group, because of their toxicological and hepatocarcinogenic effect in various susceptible animals. The toxigenicity among four AF compounds has been rated in order such as: B1 > B2 > G1 > G2. Chemically, AFs are polycyclic unsaturated compounds consisting of a coumarin nucleus flanked by a highly reactive bifuran system on one side and either a pentanone or a six member lactone on the other side. The toxic nature of AFs is due to its chemical structure. The lactone ring undergoes epoxidation to produce AFB1 2-3 epoxide, which accounts for its toxic properties. Any alteration in opening of lactone ring or saturation of double bond associated with lactone ring causes reduction in the toxicity [5]. Consumption of AF contaminated agricultural stuffs thus becomes the main route of exposure in poultry. Major adverse effects of AFs are loss of appetite, decreased feed intake, poor feed utilization, immunosuppresion, decreased egg production, and increased mortality in poultry [6–8] and additionally, the suppression of immune system [9, 10]. Immunosuppressive, hepatotoxic haemorrhage [11], carcinogenic, mutagenic, growth inhibitory [12], and teratogenic [13] effects can be detected according to animal species, sex, age and aflatoxin type, exposure dose and period. The median lethal dose (LD_{50}) of AFB1 is estimated to be between 0.3 and 18 mg/kg according to the route of administration, species of animal, age, sex, and health condition. Poultry are usually more susceptible to AFs than mammals. Within poultry, ducks are most susceptible species of all, followed by the turkey poults and thereafter, the chickens. Young animals are more susceptible to AFs than matured animals. Nutritional deficiencies, especially protein and vitamin E, increase the susceptibility to AFs [14]. Decrease in nutrient absorption in broilers fed AFB1-contaminated diet is because of the effect of toxin on systemic metabolism and not an effect on digestive functionality [15, 16].

Physical, chemical, and biological methods are essential to counteract the levels of contamination of AF, already accumulated, in foods and feeds. The cost involved and reduction in nutritive value of feed are some of the constraints that limit the use of such procedures during the feed preparation. Various studies indicate that it is practically not possible to totally eliminate the molds and their toxins from the feed. Therefore, there is need to use suitable agents that are capable of binding the toxins selectively in the gut, thus limiting their bioavailability to the consumer. Further, presence of toxic residues in poultry products (egg, meat), which enters in to the food chain, may pose potential risk by their hazardous effects on the health of human beings [17]. An approach to the aflatoxin contamination problem has been to use non-nutritive and inert adsorbents in the diet to bind AF and reduce the absorption of AF from the gastrointestinal tract. Use of adsorbents such as zeolites and alluminosillicates has proven successful, but their possible interaction with feed nutrients is a cause of concern [18, 19]. Therefore, the occurrence of AF, its detection procedures in different feedstuffs and different strategies to ameliorate its effect on the performance of poultry, and the reduction of their residues in food for food safety are discussed in detail below.

2. Occurrence

Aflatoxins were first identified in early 1960s and since then have been the most studied mycotoxins. Aflatoxins (AFs) are the most commonly occurring mycotoxins that are heterocyclic compounds produced as secondary metabolites mainly by various *Aspergillus* species including *A. flavus, A.parasiticus,* and *A. nominus* [20]. The biosynthesis of AFs consists of 18 enzymatic steps with at least 25 genes responsible for producing the enzymes and regulating the biosynthetic process [21, 22]. These mycotoxins are mainly found in agricultural products in tropical and subtropical regions [23–25]. Almost all agricultural commodities will support the growth of aflatoxin-producing fungi *A. flavus, A. parasiticus*. Formation of AF can occur during the pre and post-harvest stages of food production as long as a suitable environment for mold growth is available. Optimal conditions for AF production are a water activity in excess of 0.85 (85% RH) and a temperature of 27°C, conditions that are frequently encountered in Mediterranean region. Different crops vary in their ability to support fungal colonization because of differences in the chemical composition of each commodity. The incidence and degree of AF contamination vary with seasonal and geographical factors and also with the conditions under which the crop is grown, harvested, stored, and transported [26]. Factors affecting the production and occurrence of mycotoxins in crops and the level of contamination in feed and food entail climatic conditions such as temperature, relative humidity, and agricultural operations such as usage of fungicides. Other factors include: drying, processing, handling, packaging, storage, and transport environment. Insects play an important role in contaminating the agricultural commodities through physical damage of the grains and mechanical transmission of the microorganisms [27–30]. As such, most of the cereal grains, oil seeds, and tree nuts are susceptible to fungal invasion and consequently formations of mycotoxin aflatoxin. Agricultural products such as cereal grains and forages can be polluted during pre-harvest [field period, harvest, and post-harvest (storage and transportation period)]. Maize and other grains used in poultry feed could also be infected by pathogenic molds and thereby produce aflatoxins, even when they may be destroyed at different rates during industrial processing [2, 14, 31, 32]. The fungal species can invade foods and feedstuffs depending upon the geographical and climatic conditions of a particular region. Aflatoxins are mostly expected in tropical areas where climatic conditions and storage practices are favorable to fungal growth and toxin production, whereas other mycotoxins such as ochratoxins and fumonisins are detected in moderate, subtropical and tropical locations, with zearalenone and trichothecenes forming the worldwide mycotoxins [33, 34]. Unfortunately, the food and feed contamination by AFs is a persistent problem worldwide. The outbreaks due to AFs are more prone in tropical and subtropical areas, with a few in temperate regions. Further, the Mediterranean zones have become prone to AFs contamination due to shifting in traditional occurrence areas of AFs because of climate change, namely increase in average temperature, CO_2 levels, and rainfall pattern [35]. This has led to an increased occurrence of AFs worldwide, due to increase in contamination of crops.

Aflatoxins are often present in feedstuffs and cause some adverse effects, which can range from: vomiting, weight loss, and acute necrosis of parenchyma cells to various types of carcinoma and immunosuppression in large animals, pets, and poultry birds [36, 37]. Aflatoxin B1 (AFB1), among the four major types of AFs, is the most toxic and potent carcinogen in humans and animals [38]. AFB1 causes series of pathophysiological changes in an organism such as lower growth rate, malnutrition, silenced immune response, and disturbed gastrointestinal tract. Also, AFB1 can induce various histopathological manifestations of hepatocytes such as proliferation of the bile duct, centrilobular necrosis and fatty degeneration of the hepatocytes, and hematoma [29, 39–41]. AFB1 is already reported to induce hepatocellular carcinoma in many species of animals including fishes (rainbow trout, sock eye salmon, and guppy), poultry (turkeys, ducks, and geese), non-human primates (rhesus, cynomolgus, African green, and squirrel monkeys), and rodents (rats, mice, and tree shrews) [36, 42]. In poultry, AFB1 mainly affects the liver, kidney, immune organs (spleen, bursa of fabricius, and thymus), and gastrointestinal system. Poultry industry, factually, is one of the largest, most organized, fastest-growing, and vibrant segments of agro-industries, generating direct and indirect employment and income for millions of people, in developed and developing countries [43–45]. According to an estimate by the Food and Agriculture Organization (FAO), 25% of the world's food crops are affected by mycotoxins, and the rate of mycotoxin contamination is likely to increase in line with the trend seen in preceding years [46–49]. A worldwide mycotoxin survey in 2013 revealed that 81% of around 3000 grain and feed samples analyzed had at least one mycotoxin, which was way higher than the 10-year average (from 2004 to 2013) of 76%, in a total of 25,944 samples. The most notorious mycotoxins, thus, are aflatoxins (Afs), which often result in low performance in poultry, decreased quality of egg and meat production, and then, cause significant economic losses [50–52]. In broilers, aflatoxins drastically affect almost all valuable production factors including weight gain, feed intake, and feed conversion ratio (FCR) and induce immunosuppression, which is directly related to reduced effectiveness of vaccination programs, increased risk of infectious diseases, and high mortality. In layers, aflatoxins cause the decrease in egg production, egg size, and egg quality.

Included in the text, is a tabular presentation of various feed materials/grains with mention of their aflatoxin contamination ranges along with incidence rates (**Table 1**).

Food materials	Class of aflatoxin	Incidence rate (sample size)	Detection range	Country	References
Peanut	AFB1	57 (49)	LOD to 193 μg/kg	Algeria	[53]
Maize	Aflatoxin Total	40 (270)	—	Argentina	[54]
Maize	AFB1, AFG1		0.5–49.9 μg/kg	Brazil	[55]
Peanut	AFTotal	10 (119)	0.3–100 μg/kg	Brazil	[56]
Maize	AFB1	2.3 (44)	0–148.4 μg/kg	China	[57]
Wheat and Wheat crackers	AFB1	5.6 (178)	0.03–0.12 μg/kg	China	[58]
Peanuts	AF Total	0.15 (2494)	0.06–1602.5 μg/kg	China	[59]
Maize	AFB1, AFB2, AFG1	15, 15, 5 (20)	1.9–458.2 μg/kg	Columbia	[60]
Rice	AFB1	12.5 (24)	100–200 μg/kg	Egypt	[61]
Wheat	AFB1	33.33 (36)	<LOD to 49.79 μg/kg	Egypt	[62]
Maize	AFB1, AFB2	24.6 (61)	0.02–0.19 μg/kg	Egypt	[63]
Maize	AF Total	100 (150)	20–91.04 μg/kg	Ethiopia	[64]
Sorghum	AF Total	100 (90)	<LOD to 33.10 μg/kg	Ethiopia	[65]

Food materials	Class of aflatoxin	Incidence rate (sample size)	Detection range	Country	References
Peanut and peanut cake	AF Total	32 (160 peanut) 68 (50 peanut cake)	<LOD to 2368 μg/kg <20–158 μg/kg	Ethiopia	[66]
Sesame seeds	AFB1	77.6 (30)	LOD to 14.49 μg/kg	Greece	[67]
Maize	AF Total	37.7 (326)	<LOD to 341 μg/kg	Ghana	[68]
Sorghum	AFB1	71.42 (15)	0.005–0.02 μg/kg	India	[69]
Rice	AF Total	2.3 (87)	21.581–22.989 μg/kg	India	[70]
Rice	AFB1	100 (40)	0.29–2.9 μg/kg	Iran	[71]
Maize	AF Total	75 (140)	—	Italy	[72]
Sorghum	AFB1, AFB2, AFG1, AFG2	10.81, 5.41, 18.92, 32.43 (37)	—	Kenya	[73]
Sorghum unit	AFB1, AFB2, AFG1	44, 9, 17 (45)	0.61–28.3, 0.14–2.35, 0.39–6.95 μg/kg	Namibia	[74]
Sorghum	AFB1	28.6 (146)	0.96–21.74 μg/kg	Nigeria	[75]
Rice	AF Total	36.9 (38)	00–20.2 μg/kg	Nigeria	[76]
Rice	AF Total	50 (72)	0–40 μg/kg	Pakistan	[77]
Maize	AF Total	64.6 (82)	1–17 μg/kg	Peru	[78]
Maize	AF Total	48.2 (56)	LOD to 9.14 μg/kg	Serbia	[79]
Maize	AFB1, AFB2	1 (507)	5.2 μg/kg	South Korea	[80]
Peanut	AF Total	25 (1089)	LOD to 432 μg/kg	Taiwan	[81]
Maize	AF Total	4 (1055)	7.96–163.62 μg/kg	Turkey	[82]
Wheat	AF Total	2 (141)	0.21–0.44 μg/kg	Turkey	[83]
Peanut	AF Total	84 (102)	0.2–2177.2 μg/kg	Turkey	[84]
Sorghum	AFB1	0.7 (275)	1–14 μg/kg	Uruguay	[75]

Table 1.
Surveys of food and agricultural products contaminated with aflatoxin in different locations.

3. AF-susceptible poultry species, inter and intra-species variations: current research

3.1 Genetic variation within various poultry for susceptibility to aflatoxicosis

It is now well established that susceptibility of a poultry species to aflatoxicosis is subject to variation due to underlying genetic makeup of the host. This would mean that there already exists an inter-species variation across current range of domesticated poultry species, with respect to their threshold of clinical tolerance. The global literature is now replete with multiple reports, citing how common poultry ducklings, goslings, and turkey poults are viewed as the most susceptible in contrast to female rats (too resistant), in terms of host-to-host comparison for aflatoxin metabolism within system [85–87].

Taking leads from such literature, further reports from around the globe have well indicated a definite variability among species for degree of susceptibility across species; across breeds and genetic lines. It is well determined that ducklings and turkey poultry turn out to be the most sensitive species to aflatoxins. Next are the species of goslings, quails, and pheasants, which display intermediate sensitivity, in that scale. Hearteningly, using the same yardstick, the chickens appear to be the most resistant [88] to lethality, from aflatoxin-contaminated feeds. Earlier researchers [89] have demonstrated that the chicks can tolerate up to 3 ppm AFB in the diet without showing any significant adverse effects. A separate study found out that chickens are not only highly resistant to adverse effects of AFB1, but there could still be some modest enhancement in the body weight of chickens, when exposed to aflatoxin-contaminated diets, leading to a finding that was characterized as an hormetic-type dose-response relationship [90]. The most specific and relevant study for inter-species susceptibility evaluation by [91], who have concluded that "the susceptibility-variation among five distinct species of poultry, lied in the order of ducklings > turkey poults > goslings > pheasant chicks > chickens" in decreasing order of susceptibility, among commercial poultry. This study further documented that ducklings were 5–15 times more sensitive to aflatoxin's effects than those of laying hens, with respect to productivity outputs. Further, when the laying hen strains were compared, inter se, certain strains of hens turned out to be nearly thrice more sensitive than other strains [92].

3.2 Aflatoxicosis in ducks

As the ducks appear to be the most vulnerable species to the aflatoxicosis effects, among entire domesticated poultry, a renewed emphasis is currently on to study the whole spectrum of toxicological effects resulted in the ducks, which impact the productivity in ducks.

Way back in mid-twentieth century, when the aflatoxicosis was being described in literature, just as "*Turkey-X disease*," the report of previous research workers [93] documented that toxicological impacts from aflatoxicosis (in ducks) resulted in inappetance, abnormal vocalizations, reduced growth, besides feather picking tendencies, purple discoloration of legs and feet resulting in lameness in ducklings upon feeding with AF-contaminated diets. The typical symptoms of ducklings included: ataxia, convulsions, and opisthotonos, preceding death from aflatoxicosis. Lameness, either unilateral or bilateral, as an outcome of long-term feeding of AFB1-spiked diets (@ 200 ppb for 6 weeks) to Pekin ducks was also reported [94] resulting in near condemnation of the survivor ducks as meat animals, owing to obvious reasons. The reports of Indian labs (author's own lab at ICAR-DPR) have also shown that recurrent presence of naturally arisen AFB1 (in 30–50 ppb ranges) in Pekin ducks has largely been the reason behind huge condemnation of the aflatoxicosis survivors, which not only gave rise to carcass degradation, but also affected the usual fleshing of meat-type Pekin ducks at marketable ages, say by 6–8 weeks latest [95].

Huge genetic variation with respect to morbidity and mortality of ducks on production and fitness, even at an organized farm, has been reported between breeds of domesticated ducks, in conditions of natural aflatoxicosis [96], where duck's fertility (FRT), hatchability on total set (HTES) besides survival of adult layers were significantly affected during the laying period (20–72 weeks of age), whenever the AFB1 levels breached the 10 ppb levels in the naturally stored diets. The between-breed variation with respected to survival and production drops was settled as: The susceptibility to aflatoxins was in the order: Pekins > natives > Khaki Campbells. The authors concluded that: there remained a need for an anti-toxin duck-raising strategy, which can be based on genetics and climatic factors, including a vigilant feeding and healthcare regime.

The postmortem lesions in ducks have also been detailed by many authors to detail the organ specific changes accumulated to duckling. Many authors have reported hepatitis and nephritis with enlarged and pale kidneys. As regards the chronic effects of AFB, ascitis and hydropericardium have been reported, which were accompanied by shrunken firm nodular liver; distention of the gall bladder and hemorrhages, distended abdomen due to liver tumors and secondary ascites [97, 98].

Various microscopic lesions in the liver have been reported from AFB1 by above authors, which included fatty change in hepatocytes; proliferation of bile ducts and extensive fibrosis of liver accompanied by degenerative lesions in pancreas and kidney; and typical bile duct hyperplasia [66]. Previous researchers [97] have also reported that bile duct carcinoma in Khaki Campbell ducks resulted due to impacts of aflatoxicosis. As per the studies in ducks fed (diets spiked with AF) with AFB1, both feed intake and weight gain were reduced but without affecting feed efficiency [99].

While the threshold of clinical toxicity and subclinical toxicity in ducks would normally remain a debatable subject among scientists, the cutoff levels of AFB1 in duck feeds, prescribed in South-east Asia region and that of the West (America & Europe), are likely to vary because of the biotic and abiotic ambiences prevalent in respective regions. While other researchers [100] have cited that even feeding of 300 ppb AFB1 in Pekin duckling diets, for a period of 4 weeks, the loss in weight gain was just insignificant, the Indian studies, including that of author's own lab, have suggested that as much as 10 ppb of naturally arisen AFB1 (or higher) in duckling diets could precipitate in huge morbidity and mortalities in Pekin duck stocks. However, other authors have emphasized that mortalities to the tune of 50% of most ducklings could be witnessed in both Pekin and Khaki Campbell ducks when the naturally arisen AFB1 levels hovered around 20–41 ppb during post-monsoon periods with feeds compounded with grains stored just for 6–8 months [94]. This would mean that naturally arisen AFB1 levels were indicators of rampant and conducive growth of *Aspergillus* fungi, which not only produced AFB1 in locally stored feed, but also might have supported growth of other fungi, leading to co-production of other mycotoxins possibly, with possible increase of mycotoxin cocktails.

Earlier workers reported that duck diets spiked with AFB1 up to 48 ppb actually gave rise to huge brooder-house morbidity resulting in ~20% mortality, poorer FCRs, coupled with geno-toxicities building up within the bone marrow cells of White Pekin ducks [101].

3.3 Aflatoxicosis in turkeys

As has been reported near unanimously, for inter-species susceptibility ranking in decreasing order (Ducks → Turky → Japanese Quails → Chickens) by numerous authors [88, 91, 102–105], the susceptibility profiles of Turkey fall only next to the ducks. The turkey's sensitivity to AFB1 can safely be attributed to its efficient production of AFBO within the system, which is mostly linked to the P450 enzyme that is responsible for AFB1's bioactivation and metabolism within turkey livers. The earlier work in turkey has established well that two turkey-P450 enzymes, encoded by *CYP1A5* and *CYP3A37*, are predominantly responsible for converting AFB1 into AFBO *in vitro* and *in vivo* [105, 106–108]. The complex, i.e., P450 1A5 has high affinity (high Vmax, Kcat; low Km) and catalyzes the production of both *exo*-AFBO and the detoxified metabolite AFM1 according to traditional Michaelis-Menten kinetics. The P450 3A37 is the lower affinity catalyst, exhibiting apparent subunit allostery conforming to Hill enzyme kinetics and producing *exo*-AFBO and AFQ1.

The higher sensitivity of domestic turkey to AFB1 can therefore be attributed to an unfortunate combination of efficient P450 enzymes and dysfunctional GST enzyme system of the host that allows accumulation of AFB1 adducts in the liver. In contrast, as per reports of earlier researchers [109], the effects of AFB1 exposure in North American wild turkeys were almost similar, but less severe than those encountered in domestic poultry. This differential pattern of response may obviously be reasoned out to cumulative genetic changes that might have happened during domestic selection in commercial ones, or even be, just for the wild ones belonging to totally alien genetic background compared with domestic turkey.

Now, coming to impacts of AFB1 on major production parameters of turkeys, it surely impacts the productivity negatively, causing huge economic losses for poultry industry. Dietary exposure to AFB1 led to lower weight gain and absolute body weights in both chickens and turkeys [110, 111]. Reduced feed intake and decreased efficiency of nutrient usage together, thereafter, usually contribute to impaired growth during AFB1 infections. AFB1 lowered the FCR (feed conversion ratio) causing poultry to consume more feed to produce muscle (broilers and turkeys) [8, 99, 111, 112] and eggs (layers) [113].

The initial clinical signs reported during the outbreak of "*Turkey X disease*" included anorexia and weight loss followed by depression, ataxia, and recumbency. Most affected birds used to die within a week or two. But, at the time of death, most morbid birds frequently exhibited: opisthotonos characterized by arched neck, head down back, and legs extended backward [114], and especially these symptoms when exhibited in ducks should be differentially diagnosed from that of duck viral hepatitis, another duck disease where opisthotonos remains a characteristic symptom.

At necropsy, the body condition remained generally good, but there is generalized congestion and edema in the hosts. The liver and kidney were congested, enlarged and firm, the gall bladder was full, and the duodenum remained distended with typical catarrhal content [98, 115, 116]. Along with decreased feed conversion and weight gain, reduced spontaneous activity, unsteady gait, recumbency, anemia, and death [111, 115–117].

Many researchers [118] have summarized the minimal AFB1 concentrations (threshold of AFB1) capable of exerting major effects in different poultry species, which is extracted and placed below for reference. The authors [118] reviewed the lethal thresholds of the AFB limits in feed, in different species, for which limits of hepatic impairment and loss of productivity of these species were reviewed and compiled. In this specific comparative table involving ducks, turkeys, geese, bobwhite quails, peasants beside chickens were enumerated, where the turkeys were mentioned to be the vulnerable most with 100% lethality attained in this species with just 800 ppb of AFB1. Next were the ducks with 1000 ppb, with peasants and geese all attaining lethality at ~4000 ppb, where the chickens again proved to still far from cent percent lethality at the same (4000 ppb). The turkeys again were shown up to attain hepatic impairment just at 400 ppb AFB1, followed by ducks, geese, pheasants with 500 ppb, and the least impairment shown in the chickens at a dose of 800 ppb. The authors put up a summary of 400 ppb or higher in turkeys, followed by 500 ppb in ducks, followed by chickens, and even pheasants, which showed 800 ppb and beyond at the AFB1 doses, which could pull down production. These reviews by these authors obviously brought to fore the inherent species-specific variation in AFB1 handling capacities across such widely diverse species, when the production tended to get compromised along with the hepatic impairments.

3.4 Aflatoxicosis in quails

It has been reported long back that AFB1 in quails decreased feed conversion, egg production, egg weight, hatchability besides negatively impacting exterior and interior egg quality of quail eggs to some extent [119, 120]. Studies conducted by many researchers have recorded that histopathological analysis of aflatoxin-ingested hens revealed AFB1-characteristic lesions in tissues of the liver, kidney, and intestine [121]. Aflatoxicosis was also reported in hens, and the hematological analysis showed the decreased hemoglobin content than that of the control group [122]. However, the Indian experiences from commercial propagation of Japanese quails, thus far (over last two decades), have not been that livid with respect of AF-induced drops in growth and egg production, with largely uneventful reaction from quail growers, with respect to impact of naturally arisen AF in feed, while following recommended toxin binders in quail feeds.

3.5 Aflatoxicosis and productivity losses in chickens

As regards productive performance losses, exposure to aflatoxins lowered the reproductive performance in poultry. In layers fed with AF, age of sexual maturity got increased with expected drop in egg production [113, 123]. Egg quality parameters, including total weight, shape, albumin or yolk percentage, and shell thickness in chickens and quail can be adversely affected by AFB1, although the effects were variable among studies [110, 113, 124–126]. The declines in poultry production traits are often indirect effects of AF reducing the metabolic potential of the liver. It is obvious from the fact that impaired hepatic protein production likely contributes to AF-induced changes within eggs, as the liver is the chief site of synthesis of proteins and lipids, which are incorporated into the egg yolk.

Another extensive review of the AFB1's effect on various physiological systems of the avian species has been compiled by a different group of research workers [127] in one of their monographs for postgraduate students, over recent years. These authors have detailed and cataloged almost all of the organs and systems, where AFB1-induced injurious effects have been reported. Starting from hepatoxic effects, carcinogenic effects, teratogenic effects were individually cited by the authors, in the form of a forward from <www.Poultrysite.com>. Detailed mentions of haematopoetic, neurotoxic, and immunosuppressive effects in the birds have been documented by the authors, where authors have brought together the negative effects of AFB1 in individual physiological systems, happening across the bursa, Spleen, liver, and kidneys, besides impact on nervous system in chickens, which have been vividly documented. These authors have cited the facts of non-homogeneity in body weight of birds besides negative impacts on carcass, dressed weights, and internal organs in the chickens, as the outcome of AFB1-induced negative changes in chickens [127].

4. Detection of aflatoxin in feed

4.1 Aflatoxin extraction from feed samples

The detection and quantification of AFs in feed samples need a well-organized extraction process. AFs are generally soluble in polar protic solvents, for instance, methanol, acetone, chloroform, and acetonitrile. Therefore, the extraction of aflatoxins involves the use of these solvents such as methane, acetone, or acetonitrile mixed in different ratio with small amount of water [128, 129]. AF determination based on immunoassay technique requires extraction using mixture of methanol-water (8:2) [130, 131].

The extraction of AF is followed by a cleanup step by using immunoaffinity column (IAC) chromatography [132]. The IAC employs the high specificity and reversibility of binding between an antibody and antigen to separate and purify target analytes from matrices [133]. During sample cleanup, the crude sample extract is applied to IAC containing specific antibodies to aflatoxin immobilized on a solid support such as agarose or silica. As the crude sample moves down the column, the AF binds to the antibody and so gets retained into the column. Second washing is normally required to remove the impurities and unbound proteins. This target is achieved by using appropriate buffer with proper ionic strengths. Thereafter, the AF is recovered by using solvents such as acetonitrile, which break the bond between the antibody and the aflatoxin, which are collected as the clean elutes and then quantified, separately.

4.2 Aflatoxin detection methods

The AFs have been detected in food and feed samples according to the method of Official Analytical chemists (AOAC) [134]. The most commonly used methods are based on emission and absorption characteristics such as liquid chromatography mass spectroscopy (LC-MS) [135, 136], thin layer chromatography [137], high-performance liquid chromatography (HPLC) [138], gas chromatography (GC) [139], and enzyme-linked immunosorbent assay (ELISA) [140]. However, the drawbacks of these commonly used methods are that these methods are tiresome, time-consuming and require skilled technical persons for operation. TLC has excellent sensitivities, but it requires skilled technician, pretreatment of sample, and expensive equipment [141, 142]. Further, TLC lacks precision due to accumulated errors during sample application, plate development, and interpretation. Attempts to improve TLC have emerged in to development of automated form of TLC, which is designated as high-performance thin layer chromatography (HPTLC). HPTLC method of determination of aflatoxin has overcome the errors associated with conventional TLC through automation in sample application, development, and plate interpretation. It is worthwhile to mention that currently HPTLC is one of the most efficient and precise methods in aflatoxin analysis [143, 144]. Keeping in view, the requirement of skilled operators, costs of the equipment associated with its bulkiness, and extensive sample pretreatment, the use of HPTLC has been limited to use in laboratory, and its use in field condition is impracticable. Therefore, rapid and robust methods such as polymerase chain reaction (PCR) and nondestructive methods based on fluorescence/near infrared spectroscopy (FS/NIRS) and hyper spectral imaging (HSI) have been evolved as speedy and easy detection of AFs [145]. PCR technique has also been utilized for the molecular detection of AF producing Aspergillus flavus from peanuts [146]. Likewise, the avfa, omtA, and ver-1 genes encoding the major enzymes in AF biosynthesis were utilized as target genes to analyze AFs using multiplex PCR [147]. AFs from *Aspergillus oryzae* isolated from different Korean foods were detected by using PCR, ELISA, and HPLC [148]. Hydrospectral imaging (HIS) uses the integration of both imaging and spectroscopy to record spatial and spectral characteristics of a given sample [149–152]. Visible/near-infrared (VNIR) or short-wave NIR (SWNIR) HSI techniques are feasible for the detection of AFs as well as identification of different fungal species produced in maize [153–156]. The most appropriate analytical method differs according to the nature of detected mycotoxin, e.g., for AFs, ZEN,

OTA, HPLC fluorescence, and LC-MS/MS are commonly used, while for trichothecenes, GC-MS is mainly preferred [157–162].

Aflatoxin toxicity has a potential threat to production of safe poultry products, i.e., egg and meat. This is a permanent concern for the poultry industry, which has led to development of many methodologies for its detection in feed and other products. Toxicity of aflatoxin may occur in very low concentrations; hence, very responsive and trustworthy methods of its detection are the present need for the poultry producers and other scientific organizations dealing with the poultry research. Proper sampling, homogenization, extraction, and concentration of samples are the most common steps in many analytical procedures. Detection methods can be largely classified into qualitative and quantitative ones [158, 163]. Thin layer chromatography (TLC) can be a used for preliminary test for AFs and Ochratoxins [14, 49]. Recently, for a rapid and specific screening determination of mycotoxin type, immunological methods such as enzyme-linked immunoassay (ELISA) and radioimmunoassay (RIA) are the best approaches because they depend on specific antibodies besides their relatively low cost, easy application, and their results could be comparable with those obtained by other conventional methods such as TLC and high-performance liquid chromatography (HPLC) [164–166].

A tabular presentation has been made to summarize the various aflatoxin detoxification methods reported by various research groups, with mention of their relative advantages and disadvantages (**Table 2**).

Class of detection method	Methods	Advantages	Disadvantages	References
Chromatographic based methods	HPLC	Provide accuracy, reliability and high sensitivity	Extensive sample treatment, exhaustive pre- and post-column derivation process to improve sensitivity	[167]
	TLC	Able to detect multiple metabolites in a single test and provide good level of sensitivity	Susceptible to error, need skilled operator, substantial sample treatment and costly equipment	[167]
	HPTLC GC	Sensitive, limited errors, suitable for multi-toxin detection	Non-linearity of calibration, errant responses effects from previous samples and high variability in precision	[167]
	LC	Highly sensitive and adaptable	Slow detection compared to other methods	[167]
	LC-MS/MS	Offers sensitivity, reliability and does not need the immune-affinity clean-up columns	Expensive, tiresome sample preparation, and requires highly trained and experienced operator	[168]
	UHPLC-MS/MS	Good enough for multi-contaminated sample detection, sensible, reliable with minimum use of solvent and rapid analysis	Need trained technician, expensive high matrix effect	[169]

Class of detection method	Methods	Advantages	Disadvantages	References
Immunochemical Methods	ELISA	Provides simple procedure, cheap, rapid and multi sample testing can be done simultaneously	Cross-reactivity, time consuming clean-up process	[170]
	Radio immunoassay	It offers high sensitivity, minimal matrix effect	Involves safety concerns as radioactive elements are used in assay, false-positive possibility, problems in disposal of radioactive waste materials	[171]
Spectrometric-based methods	Fourier-transform near infrared (FT-NIR) Spectrometry	Fast, environment friendly and require less skilled operator	Time-consuming calibration needed	[172]
	Laser-induced fluorescence (LIF) screening method	Suitable for samples with low levels of contamination	Limits its uses as expensive laser materials are used	[173]
	Back-light Test	Suitable for screening purposes	Possibility of false positive cases high, greater dependency on sample size and freshness of samples	[174]
	Ion mobility spectrometry (IMS)	Offer fast detection, simplicity and sensitivity	Results interpretation difficult	[175]

Table 2.
Aflatoxin detoxification methods, their advantages and disadvantages.

5. Novel strategies to reduce toxicity

Due to the soaring preponderance of AFB1 in poultry feed, several approaches are being evolved to counter or eliminate poisoning/toxicity so as to improve safety and palatability of food products. The control strategies/approaches are classified in to pre- and post-harvest techniques. Pre-harvest techniques are inclusion of genetically modified feed materials in poultry feed formulations that are resistant to *Aspergillus* infestations, climatic aggravations, management of pesticide usage, crop rotation, and timing of plantations. The post-harvest strategies include physical methods such as appropriate drying and storage of raw materials, packaging, and usage of preservatives and pesticides. These approaches act as counteractive actions to reduce the quantity of contamination that is introduced to the raw materials, which are to be included in the compounded feed of poultry. However, these approaches are not sufficient in total elimination of AF contamination. So, more post-harvest know-hows are being utilized to detoxify the contaminated feed. These are use of physical processes, chemical/biological additives to reduce or transform AFB1. All these are discussed in detail below under different headings.

5.1 Physical methods

Hand sorting by visible fungi infection is usually found to be an efficient method to reduce AFB1 in maize kernels. On the other hand, this approach is only applicable on an industrial scale using optical sorting equipment [176]. Besides, sieving can be a useful method of reducing AF poisoning as small components such as broken kernels damaged by fungi can be a source of further spoilage [177]. There is computable differentiation in the major and minor diameters, sphericities, densities of maize kernels contaminated with Aspergillus fungi, and healthy kernels without any infestation. Dehulling is also an efficient physical method of removal of AF contamination [177]. Dehulling can remove more than 90% of AF content from maize kernel [178]. The efficiency of removal of external layer of kernels can be much more visible by floating and washing techniques [176, 179, 180]. Reduction of more than ninefold of AF has been achieved by polishing of the rice kernels [181].

The raw materials should be properly dried to contain safe moisture level, i.e., cereal grains such as maize, jowar (sorghum), bajra, and wheat should not contain more than 11–12% moisture; oilseed cakes or meals such as soybean meal, ground nut cake, sunflower cake, cottonseed cake should contain 10–11% moisture; Milling by-products such as rice bran, wheat bran, etc., should not contain more than 11–12% moisture; animal protein sources such as fish meal, meat meal, etc., should not contain more than 9–10% moisture [130]. The storage godown's relative humidity also could influence the moisture content of the feed ingredients, and therefore, proper relative humidity, i.e., <60% should be maintained in the feed storage godown. The ideal temperature during storage should be <15°C. There should be proper cross ventilation in the feed godown, and feed bags should be stored in stacks, over wooden planks or stone slabs allowing a minimum air space of 10 cm from the floor and at least 2–3 feet from the wall to allow removal of moisture from the storage area [182]. The duration of storage also affects the aflatoxin content of the feed (**Table 3**) [183].

A summary on effect of storage duration triggering growth of aflatoxin (in ppb) can be checked here.

Sunlight causes photodegradation of AF leading to significant reduction in AFB1 contents in the feed. More than 60% of AF was documented to be degraded after 30 h exposure of poultry feed to sunlight [184].

In modern feed manufacturing technology, heating treatment is mostly used to degrade mycotoxin to certain extent during processing. AFs are stable at high temperature, and therefore, high heating is required to remove them quantitatively. Many research workers have demonstrated that high temperature (150–200°C) can remove significant amount of AFB_1 (an average of 79%), which is most effective at high humidity [185–188]. Microwave heating is less effective in reducing the AF contamination. The percent of

Storage duration of feed (days)	Aflatoxin content ppb	Percent positive (%)
1–5	7.9	20.5
6.10	8.0	23.4
11–15	10.7	30.0
16–20	27.9	66.7

Table 3.
Effect of storage duration on the aflatoxin content of the mixed feed.

reduction was between 22% and 32% [184]. AF content was significantly reduced in the traditional Mexico food tartilaas by microwave thermal-alkaline treatment [189].

Gamma (ϒ)-irradiation has been demonstrated for food substrates such as groundnuts, grains, soybean, and animal feed. Irradiation by ϒ-ray with high dose (60 KGy) is moderately effective with average reduction of 65% of AF [190–194]. ϒ-irradiation (at a dose level of 5–25 KGy) of chick feed reduced the AFB1 concentration by 32–42% [184].

5.2 Chemical methods

5.2.1 Acidification

Treatment of poultry feed (AF-contaminated) with citric, lactic, tartaric, and hydrochloric acid is found to be very effective in reducing the toxicity particularly when the poultry feed is soaked in acidic solution for a particular period. AF degradation can be observed in 24 h or less when the soaking is carried out at room temperature [188, 195, 196]. On the other hand, some acids such as succinic, acetic, ascorbic, and formic have marginal effect in decreasing the AFB1 toxicity. The detoxification product of AFB1 in acidic medium is AFB2a, which is very less toxic than AFB1. Treatment with citric acid reduced the AFB1 content in duckling feed remarkably, i.e., 86–92%, whereas moderate decrease of about 67% was observed with lactic acid solutions [197, 198].

5.2.2 Ammoniation

Ammoniation (or ammonization) has been used to breakdown AFB1 in an alkaline environment. This technique involves treating contaminated food with gaseous or liquid ammonia (1.5–2%) at room temperature for a time period ranging from 24 h to 15 days approximately. By following this approach, as high as 99% degradation of AF can be achieved [199–201]. Disadvantage of this technique is the requirement of complex infrastructure to conduct ammoniation process, which led to the discontinuation of this technique worldwide [202].

5.2.3 Ozonation

Ozonation is one more novel chemical method to control AF contamination during storage of grains [203]. However, other researchers reported a reduction of 86.75% AFB1 levels in wheat, when ozonolysis was used at a concentration of 6–90 mg/l for 20 min [120]. A variety of food substrates have been investigated with ozone, indicating its effectiveness in reducing the AFB1 in many feedstuffs [153–158, 204–210]. Ozone can destroy AFs efficiently (up to 66–95%) of the initial concentration in cereal grains and flours, soybean, and peanut [211–213].

5.3 Biological method

Reduction in AFB1 is observed probably due to metabolism or by physically binding of AFB1 directly when food substrates are inoculated with strains of a particular bacteria, fungi, or yeast. Two *Lactobacillus amylovorus* strains and one *Lactobacillus rhamnosus* strain removed more than 50% AFB1 rapidly after 72 h of incubation. L. *rhamnosus* strain (LC-705) can significantly and very quickly remove approximately 80% of AFB1 from culture media, which is dependent on temperature as well as concentration of the bacteria [214]. The GG strain of *L.rhamnosus* reduced the AFB1 contamination by 54% in the soluble fraction of the luminal fluid within a time of 1 min compared with *L. rhamnosus* LC-705, which removed 44% AFB1 under similar conditions [215]. There was 72% reduction in uptake of AFB1 by the intestinal tissue in presence of *L. rhamnosus* strain GG compared with 63% and 37% by *Propionibacterium freudenreichi spp*. *Shermanii JS* and *L. rhamnosus* strain LC-705, respectively. AFB1 degradation as high as 80% has been reported by using several genera of bacteria, yeast, and fungi such as *Lactobacillus*, *Saccharomyces*, *Cellulomicrobium,* and *Pleurotuseryngii* with treatment time up to several days [216–221]. Addition of *Saccharomyces cerevisiae* CECT strain to drinking water of broilers fed AFB1-contaminated diet (1.2 mg/kg) resulted in significant improvement related to production and biochemical parameters, hepatotoxicity, and histopathology of liver [222]. Fungal strains such as Aspergillus niger, Eurotiumherbariorum, a Rhizopus spp., and non-aflatoxin producing *A.flavus* were able to convert AFB1 to aflatoxicol-A (AFL-A); and then AFA-L was converted to aflatoxicol-B (AFL-B) by the actions of organic acids produced from the fungi. These AFA-A and AFA-L compounds are nontoxic indicating the significant role of fungi in detoxifying AFB1. Rhizopus oligosporus was able to inhibit or to degrade AFB1 when cultured together with AFB1-producing fungi *A.flavus* [223]. Botanical extracts such as aqueous extracts of various plants species to dissolve AFB1 have been studied to determine percent degradation after incubating the toxin in this aqueous extract for a time period of 24–72 h. The extracts from Adhatodavasica Ness and Corymbiacitridora achieved >95% degradation of AFB1 [224–227]. However, active components in these plant extracts responsible for this degradation need to be identified, which could prove useful for increasing the efficiency of this method of reduction of AFB1 in poultry feed. The potential of purified enzymes from various biological sources has been investigated for AFB1 degradation. These enzymes are laccases, manganese peroxidase, and Bacillus aflatoxin-degrading enzyme. The efficacy of this strategy is very high, but they have not been tested on food substrates, so the efficacy on food products is still unknown [202]. The time of enzyme treatment is high, which may take several days to complete the process. Therefore, this method may not be practicable for large-scale applications [228–231].

5.4 Nutritional supplements method

A number of feed supplements have provided protection against the damage caused by AFB1. Fat-soluble vitamins such as vitamin A, E, K, and D could be used in preventing the toxic effect of aflatoxins [232]. Supplementation of vitamins A, E, and C has resulted in enhanced antioxidative effect in poultry birds and protects the immune cells from oxidative damage induced by AFB1 [233]. Many studies conducted worldwide have been compiled together in a broad meta-analysis in poultry, where the nutritional supplements are exploited against AFB1 in broilers, and some of them could be well deliberated as well organized and useful to improve the adverse effects ofAFB1 [234]. Selenium (Se) and zinc (Zn) are two understudied trace elements for their protective roles against oxidative stresses and other adverse effects induced by AFB1. A number of studies have documented the importance of Se and Zn in human and animal biology when used optimally. Selenium is an essential nutrient of fundamental importance inhuman and animal biology. Se is a significant feed-derived natural antioxidant in poultry, and adequate level of Se is crucial for chicken health, productive and reproductive characteristics (embryonic development and sperm quality), and optimal functioning of immune system [235]. Two major Se sources, which are inorganic (selenite orselenate) and organic selenium (seleno-methionine), are used in poultry [236]. AFB1 exposure induced liver dysfunction by disturbing the tissue enzyme activity and enhanced apoptosis, but the Se administration protected liver tissues against AFB1-induced toxicity [237]. A number of studies conducted on various organs in poultry birds demonstrated the protective effects of Se against AFB1 [238–240]. The dietary sodium selenite in the feed of broiler has excellent effects on oxidative stress and apoptosis and can amend the immunosuppression effects induced by AFB1 in spleen of broiler [239]. Se supplementation has improved AFB1-induced apoptosis at a concentration of 0.4 mg/kg [240]. Further, Se supplementation in broiler diet provided protection against AFB1-induced changes in the ileum, and sodium selenite improved the cellular immune functioning of the AFB1-affected ileum mucosa [238]. Se inhibits AFB1-DNA binding and adducts formation and sodium selenite and Se-enriched yeast extract protect cells from AFB1 cytotoxicity [241]. Out of all the functions, antioxidant and anti-tumor abilities are the most important roles played by Se. Se may prevent the binding of DNA with carcinogens as well as reactive Se metabolites can render the carcinogens into non-carcinogenic compounds. Dietary Se has been shown to protect chicks from AFB1-induced liver injury by inhibiting CYP450-enzyme, which is responsible for the activation of AFB1 to toxic AFBO [242]. Zinc (Zn) is known for its beneficial effects on humans and animals for many decades due to its principal role in individual's growth, development, and optimal functioning of various physiological processes. Certainly, the past two decades have seen a fast growth in knowledge of the fundamental mechanisms, whereby Zn put forth its universal effects on immune function, disease resistance, and general health [243–245]. Although a number of studies have been carried out on AF-induced systemic toxicity in poultry, signifying protective effects of zinc against a range of noxious agents in human and different laboratory animal [246–249]. Only few studies focused on defensive effects of Zn against AFB1. Zn supplementation in AFB1-intoxicated birds significantly enhanced the growth performance of poultry birds in terms of higher body weight gain and better feed efficiency [250]. The function of Zn in enhancing various systems of the body could be used as modifying means against AFB1 intoxication.

5.5 Addition of adsorbents method

The best way to neutralize aflatoxins already present in feed is by binding them to an inert compound before they are absorbed from the intestine. One of the methods of detoxification of aflatoxin is the use of non-nutritive adsorptive materials in the diet to reduce aflatoxin absorption from the gastrointestinal tract. When an adsorbent is added to the feed, it adsorbs the aflatoxins in the gastrointestinal tract (GIT) and safely excretes in the feces; and thereby it prevents absorption and transport to the target organs. Hence, the final effect of addition of adsorbent is reduction in the dose of absorbable toxin to a concentration that does not affect the performance adversely. The use of activated charcoal as an oral remedy for the management of toxicity is well recognized. Charcoal acts as an insoluble carrier that non-specifically adsorbs molecules, thereby preventing their absorption [251]. The efficacy of activated charcoal in binding AF has been demonstrated by many research workers [252–255]. Addition of 200 ppm of activated charcoal to broiler diet contaminated with 0.5 ppm aflatoxin provided protection to broilers against harmful effects of AF on performance and biochemical parameters [256]. Dietary addition of super-activated charcoal @ 0.5% was marginally effective in ameliorating some of the toxic effects associated with AF, i.e., diet contaminated with 4 mg AF [251]. Addition of esterified glucomannan

(EGM) in broiler diet significantly decreased the harmful effect of AF contamination (300 ppb) [257]. Dietary supplementation of esterified glucomannan (0.05%) was effective in ameliorating the toxicity of naturally contaminated diet containing Aflatoxin 168 ppb, ochratoxin 8.4 ppb, zearalenone 54 ppb, and T-2 toxin 32 ppb [258]. Dietary addition of super-activated charcoal (SAC) @ 0.5% of diet was marginally effective in counteracting the toxic effects associated with chronic toxicosis in growing broilers. The protective effect probably involves the sequestration of the toxic molecules in the gastrointestinal tract and chemisorptions to the charcoal, which suggests that SAC is highly variable in its ability to ameliorate the toxic effects of AF in growing broilers and to bind AF in *vivo* [251]. The weight of broilers increased by 63–100% by addition of activated charcoal, bentonite, and fuller's earth to aflatoxin-contaminated feed (120 μg/kg feed). However, bentonite addition was more effective in counteracting histopathological effects compared with activated charcoal and fuller's earth [259]. A commercial binder, which is an extra-purified clay containing diatomaceous earth mineral, antioxidants curcuminoids extracted from turmeric and enzymes (Epoxidase and esterase), was added @ 0.2% to broiler chicken diet contaminated with 0.6 ppm AFB1. The addition of binder could significantly counter the harmful effects (depressed body weight, increased feed intake, and poor FCR). On the other hand, the beneficial effect on nutrient digestibility and gut function of broilers does not get confirmed [260]. Supplementation of diatomaceous earth, sodium bentonite, and zeolite at level of 0.5% or 1% individually or in combination to a 300 ppm aflatoxin B1-contaminated broiler feed was effective in improving the harmful effects of aflatoxin toxicity on the liver and livability percentage in broiler chicks. Nonetheless, sodium bentonite and zeolite were more efficient than diatomaceous earth in ameliorating the toxicity [261]. Efficacy of sodium calcium allumino-silicate, curcumin derived from turmeric (Curcuma longa), and sodium bentonite has been proven beneficial in ameliorating the adverse effects of AF on broiler chicks and growing poultry [262–265].

Further, a summary of various studies employing different detoxification methods to control aflatoxin is placed in the cited table for ease of interpretation, with relevant references (**Table 4**).

5.6 Emerging novel approaches to overcome aflatoxicosis: Genetics vs epigenetics

Genetic approaches to control aflatoxicosis can be straightforward, which can rely on a genetic selection to bring in tolerance in the host (poultry) to moderate or high levels of dietary aflatoxins. The experiences available at the ICAR's duck research and breeding facility at Bhubaneswar, India, provide some promising trends in this direction. The primary breed and strain differences evident in ducks (CARI, RC's studies) do sustain a promise that through long-term selection program or by prudent cross-breedings, the commercial ducks could be rendered tolerant to moderate dietary aflatoxins (40–50 ppb levels), as the native ducks are seen to tolerate such sporadic toxin spurts, better than Khaki Campbells and White Pekins [64], without exhibiting much morbidities in layers. However, both ethics and practicality could discourage such a selective breeding approach against aflatoxicosis, unless safeguards are in place to prevent significant residues generated within the birds from spiking of their diets with AFs, from being passed on to any of the public food chain, through landing of such genetic stocks in the consumer market inadvertently.

Marks and Wyatt (1980) were the first such team of workers [270] who have observed different mortality patterns resulting from acute aflatoxicosis in various

Detoxification method	Specific agent used	Amount of agent	% Reduction in AFB1	Initial Amount of AFB1 (ng/g)	Substrate	Treatment Time (min)	References
1. Physical method	Heat	200°C	97	100.2	Wheat	30	[186]
a. Temperature	Heat	150°C	81.2	10	Soybeans	90	[188]
	Heat	150°C	78.4	237	Peanuts	120	[185]
b. Irradiation	ϒ-irradiation	25 kGy	42.7	192.1–894	Chick feed	-	[135]
	ϒ-irradiation	15 kGy	18.2	25	Poultry feed mix.	-	[190, 191]
	ϒ-irradiation	8 kGy	60.26	50.38	maize	-	[194]
c. Organism	Lactobacillus rhamnosus	$2.5X10^{10}$ CFU/ml	71	10 ng/ml	Aqueous solution	-	[219]
			29.9–44.5	50–500 ng/g		-	[221]
	L. plantarum	10^8 CFU/ml	93.12	50 ng/ml	Maize	72 h	[218]
	L.acidophilus	$7X10^9$ CFU/ml	86	128 ng/g	Cereal	28 days	[216]
	Pleurotus eryngii	3 g			maize		
2. Chemical method	Citric acid	1 N	97.22	4–30 ng/g	Rice	15 min	[196]
a. Acidification	Citric acid	1 N	94.1	7.6 ng/g	Soybean	18 h	[188]
	Acetic acid	1 M	12.5	200 ng/ml	Aqueous solution	24 h	[195]
b. Ammoniation	Ammonia	1.50%	99.3	750 ng/g	Maize	13 days	[199]
	Ammonia	2.00%	52.7–67.7	17–7500 ng/g	Maize	60 min	[201]
	Ammonia	2.00%	88.02	4000 ng/g	Maize	24 h	[200]
c. Ozonation	Ozone	40 ppm	86.75	10 ng/g	Wheat	20 min	[204]
	Ozone	21 mg/l	25	180 ng/g	Peanuts	96 h	[206]
	Ozone	50 mg/l	89.4	189.53 ng/g	Peanuts	60 h	[207]
	Ozone	75 mg/l	78.8	53.6 ng/g	Cornflour	60 min	[209, 210]
	Ozone	90 mg/l	88.1	83 ng/g	Maize	40 min	[209, 210]
	Ozone	60 mg/l	65.9	200 ng/g	peanuts	30 min	[205]
3. Combination of methods	ammonia + heat	2% ammonia + 121°C	99	17–7500 ng/g	Maize	120 min	[201]
a. Ammoniation + heat	ammonia + heat	2% ammonia + 121°C	99.9	4000 ng/g	Maize	15 min	[200]
c. Alkalization + heat	NaOH + heat	NaOH to PH 10 + 98°C	97	34.50 ng/g	Dried fig	60 min	[266]

DOI: http://dx.doi.org/10.5772/intechopen.107438

Detoxification method	Specific agent used	Amount of agent	% Reduction in AFB1	Initial Amount of AFB1 (ng/g)	Substrate	Treatment Time (min)	References
d. Acidification + heat	HCl + heat	5 M HCl + 110°C	100	45.68 ng/g	Maize	4 h	[267]
	Lactic acid + heat	1 M Lactic acid + 80°C	85.1	1000 ng/g	Aqueous solution	120 m	[268]
	Citric acid + heat	0.1 g/ml citric acid + 120°C	93.1	383 ng/g	pistachios	60 min	[269]

Table 4.
Summary of studies using various detoxification methods to degrade AFB1.

growth-selected lines of Japanese quails of USDA experimental facilities in 1980s. This observation had thereafter led to the genetic selection of Japanese quails for resistance to acute aflatoxicosis by breeding survivors from a population of quails, which were given a single oral dose of aflatoxin that resulted in high mortality [271]. After five generations of selection, an 11-fold increase in resistance was attained in one of the aflatoxin-resistant lines. The next group of workers observed genetic variation in certain physiological parameters of selected commercial broiler populations and suggested the feasibility of genetic selection of chickens for infusing resistance to aflatoxicosis [272]. Many other researchers had observed genetic variation in a non-selected population of chickens [273].

The other successful directional selective breeding for AFB1 resistance was also reported [274]. Under their breeding trials, two populations of broiler chickens [Athens-Canadian (AC) versus another broiler commercial stock] were subjected to genetic selection for resistance to aflatoxicosis by exposing the respective chickens from each of the stocks (two) with a single oral dose of aflatoxin, which was capable of resulting in 40–70% mortality, otherwise. A simultaneous, non-selected control group was also maintained, which was not exposed to any AFB1. As for the selection method, the birds surviving the aflatoxin challenge were propagated as breeders, for subsequent generations. According to the outcome of their study, rapid progress was visible within the AC population for resistance to aflatoxin, whereas only moderate progress for AFB1 resistance was attained in the commercial broiler stock. After five generations of selection in the AC population, LD50 values of 9.42 and 17.05 milligrams aflatoxin per kg body weight (BW) were determined for both the non-selected and selected lines. Similarly, after four such generations of such selection in above commercial broiler population, LD50 values of 6.05 and 8.02 mg aflatoxin/kg BW were determined for the non-selected and selected lines, respectively. These experiments demonstrated that genetic progress for AFB1 tolerance could be achievable in chickens, but the quantum of such progress for resistance to AFB1 could be influenced by the population's background, meaning response to such genetic selection for such AFB1 resistance or tolerance was always a subject of genetic constitution of the hosts.

On a practical front, there have been couple of studies that attempted direct breeding of ducks for tolerance or resistance to AFB1's presence in diets, on selective-breeding platforms, way back in 1980s, after which very little progress has been registered in duck-producing countries. The obvious interpretation could be that ensuring a diet with minimal cutoff levels for AFB1, which was achievable using toxin binders, mold inhibitors, etc., was probably preferred to (better than) raising stocks with resistance to AFB1.

5.6.1 Epigenetic studies on aflatoxicosis

Epigenetics is the study of heritable phenotypic alterations caused due to change in chromosomal topology rather than change in DNA sequence [275, 276]. The underlying epigenetic processes such as chromatin remodeling, non-coding RNAs (micro RNAs), DNA methylation, acetylation, deacetylation, histone modification, etc., are affected by prolonged exposure to aflatoxin, causing alteration in protein synthesis and thereby the gene expressions. Aflatoxin-B1 mainly induces DNA methylation, which plays a critical role in the development of all most all cancer types owing to its silencing effect on tumor suppressor genes [277]. In this process, the fifth carbon of the cytosine in dinucleotide 5'-CG-3′ is selectively methylated to form 5-mC [278, 279]. Aberrant methylation of promoters in eukaryotic cell may lead to silencing of regulatory genes especially tumor suppressor genes and thereafter, affect their signal pathways and lead to development of disease and cancers. Alteration in cellular epigenome compromises genomic stability and alters gene expression, which thereby affect the central dogma of molecular biology and ultimately phenotypic characters.

Few human studies have been reported in literature detailing the epigenetic changes which accompany aflatoxin-exposure, across various vital organs such as white blood cells, egg yolk, plasma, etc. It has been reported that maternal exposure to aflatoxin during early embryonic development leads to formation of aflatoxin albumin (AF-alb) adducts and genome-wide differential DNA methylation patterns of white blood cells for 71 CpG sites, including in genes related to growth and immune function [280]. It has been reported to cause various types of cancers such as colon cancer [281], sarcomas [282], lung cancer [283], ovarian cancer [284], leukemia [285], urological cancer [286], breast cancer [287], Hodgkin lymphoma [288], including cardiovascular diseases [289] and schizophrenia [290].

Though epigenetic approaches raise hopes for a long-term strategy to overcome aflatoxicosis problems in ducks, the literature is just hollow, except some rudimentary reports. The ICAR-DPR's own annual report [95] indicated that most significant aflatoxicosis-induced production losses peaked and precipitated only in alternate generations/years, despite emergence of naturally arisen dietary aflatoxins (10–50 ppb ranges throughout the year) since last decade, which suggest that epigenetic sensitization of the ducklings/ducks every generation at early or perinatal stages, which are usually the phases of methylation-induction processes in an epigenetic regime. The RC, CARI (now a regional Station of Directorate on Poultry, Research, Bhubaneswar, India) has just concluded a large-funded program on epigenetics research in ducks, which has shown positive feedbacks through better egg-production recorded from AF-sensitized ducks versus the controls, thus signifying feasibility of such approaches in coming decades.

6. Conclusions

Almost all classes of poultry are physiologically vulnerable and susceptible to aflatoxins, especially the AFB1, which produces acute, chronic, mutagenic, and teratogenic toxicity along with causing millions of dollars per year damage to the poultry industry, worldwide. The high frequency and levels of AFB1 recently found in food supplies, particularly, poultry feed of various countries indicate wide exposure of poultry birds to this toxin, which still remain uncontrolled. The most appropriate analytical method differs according to the nature of detected mycotoxin, e.g., for AFs, ZEN, OTA, HPLC fluorescence, and LC-MS/MS are commonly used, while for trichothecenes, GC-MS is mainly preferred. Due to the increasing abundance of AFB1 in poultry feed, several approaches are being evolved to counter or eliminate poisoning/toxicity so as to improve safety and palatability of food products. Between pre- and post-harvest strategies, there are many options available to reduce the toxicity to a great extent. Large-scale implementation of these techniques could make a large impact worldwide to reduce the aflatoxin related toxicities such as growth impairment, histopathology of organs, and immunosuppression in poultry birds. Development of suitable method for detection of aflatoxin in field level and environment-friendly detoxification keeping in view the food safety will be beneficial strategies for achievement of poultry products, which will be safe and secured for human consumption. Quality control of feed ingredients; prevention of fungal growth with reduction in concomitant aflatoxin production; use of efficient detection method and suitable environment-friendly detoxification methods, are essential to the feed manufacturers to reduce the exposure to aflatoxin and to make the poultry production a profitable enterprise. Among various classes of AFB1-susceptible poultry species, recent research on epigenetics in ducks has shown some positive feedbacks regarding feasibility of such approaches in upcoming decades, while needs to develop poultry species genetically resistant to Aflatoxins through direct selection may not find a great favor from primary breeders anymore, in twenty-first century despite promising results documented during late-twentieth century.

Author details

Surya Kanta Mishra* and Bijaya Kumar Swain
ICAR-Directorate of Poultry Research Regional Station, Bhubaneswar, Odisha, India

*Address all correspondence to: suryakmishra@yahoo.com

References

[1] Jewers K. Mycotoxins and their Effect on Poultry Production. Options Mediterrraneenenes. 1990;**7**:195-202. Available from: https://en-ergomix.com/mycotoxins/articles/mycotoxins-their-effect-poultry-33370.htm/07/15/22

[2] Reddy KRN, Salleh B, Saad B, Abbas HK, Abel CA, Shier WT. An overview of mycotoxin contamination in foods and implications for human health. Toxin Reviews. 2010;**29**:3-26

[3] Gupta RC. Aflatoxins, ochratoxins and citrinin. In: Reproductive and Developmental Toxicology (Ed. R.C. Gupta), Burlington, MA, USA: Elsevier; 2011. pp. 753-763

[4] Womack EDW, Brown AE, Sparks DL. A recent review of non-biological remediation of aflatoxin-contaminated crops. Journal of The Science of Food and Agriculture. 2014;**94**:1706-1714

[5] Johri TS. Mycotoxins in feed and feeding of animals. In: Nutrient and Dietetics under Clinico-therapeutic Conditions of Pet and Farm Animals, March 20–April 18, 2001. IVRI, Izatnagar, India: CAS in Animal Nutrition; 2001

[6] Miazzo R, Rosa CA, Carvalho De Queiroz EC, Magnoli C, Chiacchiera SM, Palacio G, et al. Efficacy of synthetic zeolite to reduce the toxicity of aflatoxin in broiler chicks. Poultry Science. 2000;**79**:1-6

[7] Verma J, Johri TS, Swain BK. Effect of varying levels of aflatoxin, ochratoxin and their combinations on the performance and egg quality characteristics in laying hens. Asian Australasian Journal of Animal Sciences. 2003;**16**(7):1015-1019

[8] Verma J, Johri TS, Swain BK, Amina S. Effect of graded levels of aflatoxin, ochratoxin and their combinations on the performance and immune response of broilers. British Poultry Science. 2004;**45**:512-518

[9] Gabal MA, Azzam AH. Interaction of AF in the feed immunization against selected infectious diseases in poultry. II. Effect on one-day-old layer chicks simultaneously vaccinated against Newcastle disease, infectious bronchitis and infectious bursal disease. Avian Pathology. 1998;**27**:290-295

[10] Oguz H, Hadimli HH, Kurtoglu V, Erganis O. Evaluation of humoral immunity of broilers during chronic AF (50 and 100 ppb) and CLI exposure. Research in Veterinary Science. 2003;**154**:483-486

[11] Ortatatli M, Oguz H. Ameliorative effects of dietary CLI on pathological changes in broiler chickens during aflatoxicosis. Research in Veterinary Science. 2001;**71**:59-66

[12] Oguz H, Kurtoglu V. Effect of clinoptilolite on fattening performance of broiler chickens during experimental aflatoxicosis. British Poultry Science. 2000;**41**:512-517

[13] Sur E, Celik I. Effects of aflatoxin B1 on the development of bursa of fabricius and blood lymphocyte acid phosphatases of the chicken. British Poultry Science. 2003;**44**:558-566

[14] Bryden WL. Mycotoxins: Natural Food Chain Contaminants and Human Health. Gatton, QLD, Australia. Burlington, MA, USA: Elsevier: University of Queensland; 2011

[15] Verma J, Swain BK, Johri TS. Effect of various levels of aflatoxin and ochratoxin A and combinations thereof on protein

and energy utilization in broilers. Journal of the Science of Food and Agriculture. 2002;**87**(5):1412-1417

[16] Verma J, Johri TS, Swain BK. Effect of aflatoxin, ochratoxin and their combination on protein and energy utilization in white leghorn laying hens. Journal of the Science of Food and Agriculture. 2007;**87**:760-764

[17] Patil RD, Sharma R, Arsani RK. Mycotoxicosis and its control in poultry: A review. Journal of Poultry Science Technology. 2014;**2**:1-10

[18] Phillips TD. Dietary clay in the chemo prevention of AF-induced diseases. Toxicology Letters. 1999;**52**(Supplement):118-126

[19] Rosa CAR, Miazzo R, Magnoli C, Salvano M, Chiacchiera SM, Ferrero S, et al. Evaluation of the efficacy of bentonite from the south of Argentina to ameliorate the toxic effects of AF in broilers. Poultry Science. 2001;**80**:139-144

[20] Kutzman CP, Horn BW, Hesseltine CW. *Aspergillus nomius*, a new–aflatoxin producing species related to *aspergillus flavus* and *aspergillus tamari*. Antonie Leeuwenhoek. 1987;**53**:147-158

[21] Yu J, Bhatnagar D, Erlich KC. Aflatoxin biosynthesis. Review iberoam, Micology. 2002;**19**:191-200

[22] Yabe K, Nakajima H. Enzyme reactions and genes in aflatoxin biosynthesis. Applied Microbiology and Biotechnology. 2004;**64**:745-755

[23] Leszczynska J, Kucharska U, Zegota H. Aflatoxins in nuts assayed by immunological methods. European Food Research and Technology. 2000;**210**(3):213-215

[24] Wu HC, Santella R. The role of aflatoxins in hepatocellular carcinoma. Hepatitis Monthly. 2012;**12**(10 HCC):e7238

[25] Da Rocha MEB, Freire FCO, Maia FEF, MIF G, Rondina D. Mycotoxins and their effects on human and animal health. Food Control. 2014;**36**(1): 159-165

[26] Jewers K, Coker RD, Blunden G, Jazwinski MJ, Sharkey AJ. Problems involved in the determination of aflatoxin levels in bulk commodities. International Biodeterioration. 1986;**22S**:83-88

[27] Chrevatidis A. Mycotoxins/ occurrence and determination. In: Caballero B, editor. Encyclopedia of Food Science and Nutrition. 2nd ed. Oxford, UK: Academic Press; 2003. pp. 4089-4096

[28] Abbas HK, Cartwright RD, Weiping Xie W, Shier WT. Aflatoxin and fumonisin contamination of corn (maize, *Zea mays*) n hybrids in Arkansas. Crop Prtection. 2006;**25**:1-9

[29] Richard JL. Some major mycotoxins and their mycotoxicoses—An overview. International Journal of Food Microbiology. 2007;**119**(1):3-10

[30] Marroquin-Cardona AG, Johnson NM, Phillips TD, Hayes AW. Mycotoxin in a changing global environment—A review. Food and Chemical Technology. 2014;**69**:220-230

[31] Griessler K, Rodrigues I, Handl J, Hofstetter U. Occurrence of mycotoxins in southern Europe. World Mycotoxin Journal. 2010;**3**:301-309

[32] Kocasari FS, Mor F, Oguz MN, Oguz FK. Occurrence of mycotoxins in feed samples in Burdur Province,

Turkey. Environmental Monitoring and Assessment. 2013;**185**:4943-4949

[33] Sweeny MJ, ADW D. Mycotoxin production by *Aspergillous*, *fusarium* and *Pencillium* species. International Journal of Food Microbiology. 1998;**43**:141-158

[34] Afsah-Hejri L, Jinap S, Hajeb P, Radu S, Shakibazadeh S. A review on mycotoxin in food and feed: Malaysia case study. Comprehensive Reviews in Food Science and Food Safety. 2013;**12**:629-651

[35] WFO M, WCA G, Shephard GS, Vismar HF. Mycotoxins: A Global Problem. Mycotoxins: Detection Methods, Management, Public Health and Agricultural Trade. 4th ed. Oxford: CABI; 2008. pp. 29-39

[36] Robens J, Richard J. Aflatoxins in animal and humanhealth. In: Reviews of Environmental Contamination and Toxicology. New York: Springer Verlag Inc; 1992. pp. 69-94

[37] Bbosa GS, Kitya D, Odda J, Ogwal-Okeng J. Aflatoxins metabolism, effects on epigenetic mechanisms and their role in carcinogenesis. Health. 2013;**5**(10A):14-34

[38] Guzman de Pena D. Exposure to aflatoxin B1 in experimental animals and its public health significance. Salud Publica de Mexico. 1975;**49**(3):227-235

[39] Ellis W, Smith J, Simpson B, Oldham J, Scott PM. Aflatoxins in food: Occurrence, biosynthesis, effects on organisms, detection, and methods of control. Critical Reviews in Food Science & Nutrition. 1991;**30**(4):403-439

[40] Iheshiulor O, Esonu B, Chuwuka O, Omede A, Okoli I, OgbuewuI. Effects of mycotoxins in animal nutrition: A review. Asian Journal of Anim Sciences. 2011;**5**:19-33

[41] Abrar M, Anjum FM, Butt MS, Pasha I, Randhawa MA, Saeed F, et al. Aflatoxins: Biosynthesis, occurrence, toxicity, and remedies. Critical Review in Food Science and Nutrition. 2013;**53**(8):862-874

[42] Wogan GN. Aflatoxins as risk factors for hepatocellularcarcinoma in humans. Cancer Research. 1992;**52**(Suppl. 7): 2114s-2118s

[43] Blake DP, Tomley FM. Securing poultry production fromthe ever-present Eimeria challenge. Trends in Parasitology. 2014;**30**(1):12-19

[44] Islam MK, Forhad UM, Alam MM. Challenges and prospects of poultry industry in Bangladesh. European Journal of Business and Management. 2014;**6**(7):116-127

[45] Windhorst HW. Changes in poultry production and trade worldwide. World's Poultry Science Journal. 2006;**62**(04):585-602

[46] Dalcero A, Magnoli C, Chiacchiera S, Palacios G, Reynoso M. Mycoflora and incidence of aflatoxin B1, zearalenone and deoxynivalenol in poultry feeds in Argentina. Mycopathologica. 1997;**137**(3):179-184

[47] Shetty PH, Bhatt RV. Natural occurrence of fumonisin B1 and its co-occurrence with aflatoxin B1 in Indian sorghum, maize, and poultry feeds. Journal of Agriculture and Food Chemistry. 1997;**45**(6):2170-2173

[48] Fraga M, Curvello F, Gatti M, Cavaglieri L, Dalcero A, da Rocha RC. Potential aflatoxin and ochratoxin A production by aspergillus species in poultry

feed processing. Veterinary Research Communication. 2007;**31**(3):343-353

[49] Zinedine A, Juan C, Soriano J, Molto J, Idrisi L, Manes J. Limited survey for the occurrence of aflatoxins in cereals and poultry feeds from Rabat. Morocco. International Journal of Food Microbiology. 2007;**115**(1):124-127

[50] Bintvihok A, Thiengnin S, Doi K, Kumagai S. Residue of aflatoxins in the liver, muscle and eggs of domestic fowls. Journal of veterinary and medical. Science. 2002;**64**(11):1037-1039

[51] Fink-Gremmels J, Malekinejad H. Clinical effects and biochemical mechanisms associated with exposure to the myco estrogen zearalenone. Animal Feed Science and Technology. 2007;**137**(3):326-341

[52] Lizarraga-Paulin EG, Moreno-Martinez E, Miranda-Castro SP. Aflatoxins and Their Impact on Human and Animal Health: An Emerging Problem. In: Ramon G, Gonzalez G, editor. Universidad, Autonoma de occidente, Colombia. InTech Open Access Publisher; 2011

[53] Ait Mimoune N, Arroyo-Manzanares N, Gamiz-Gracia L, Garcia-Campana AM, Bouti K, Sabaou N, et al. Aspegillus section Flavi and aflatoxins in dried figs and nuts in Algeria. Food Additives and Contaminants Part B. 2018;**11**(2):119-125

[54] Castellari CC, Cendoya MG, Marcos FV, Barrera V, Pacin AM. Extrinsic and intrinsic factors associated with mycotoxigenic fungi populations of maize grains (*Zea mays* L.) stored in silo bags in Argentina. Revista Argentina de Microbiologia. 2015;**47**(4):350-359

[55] Oliveira MS, Rocha A, Sulyok M, Krska R, Mallmann CA. Natural mycotoxin contamination of maize (*Zea mays* L.) in the south region of Brazil. Food Control. 2017;**73**:127-132

[56] Martins LM, Sant'Ana AS, FungaroMHP, SilvaJJ, doNascimentoMDS, Frisvad JC, et al. The biodiversity of aspergillus section Flavi and aflatoxins in the Brazillian peanut production chain. Food Research International. 2017;**94**(4):101-107

[57] Xing F, Liu X, Wang L, Selvaraj JN, Jin N, Wang Y, et al. Distribution and variation of fungi and major mycotoxins in pre- and post-nature drying maize in North China plain. Food Control. 2017;**80**:244-251

[58] Zhao Y, Wang Q, Huang J, Ma L, Chen Z, Wang F. Aflatoxin B1 and sterigmatocystin in wheat and wheat products from supermarkets in China. Food Additives and Contaminants: Part B. 2018;**11**(1):9-14

[59] Wu L, Ding X, Li P, Du X, Zhou H, Bai YZ, et al. Aflatoxin contamination of peanuts at harvest in China from 2010 to 2013 and its relationship with climatic conditions. Food Control. 2016;**60**:117-123

[60] Diaz GJ, Krska R, Sulyok M. Mycotoxins and cyanogenic glycosides in staple foods of three indigenous people of Colombian Amazon. Food Additives and Contaminants: Part B. 2015;**8**(4):291-297

[61] Moharram A, Yasser M, Sayed M, Omar O, Idres M. Mycobiota and mycotoxins contaminating rice grains in EI-Minia, governorate, Egypt. Biosciences Biotechnology Research Asia. 2019;**16**(1):167-178

[62] Hathout AS, Abel-Fattah SM, Abou-Sree YH, Fouzy AS. Incidence and exposure assessment of aflatoxins and ochratoxin A in Egyptian wheat. Toxicology Reports. 2020;**7**:867-873

[63] Abdallah MF, Girgin G, Baydar T. Mycotoxin detection in maize, commercial feed, and raw dairy Milk samples from Assiut City, Egypt. Veterinary Science. 2019;**6**(2):57

[64] Chauhan NM, Washe AP, Minota T. Fungal infection and aflatoxin contamination in maize collected from Gedeo zone, Ethiopia. Springer Plus. 2016;**5**(1):753

[65] Taye W, Ayalew A, Chala A, Dejene M. Aflatoxin B1 and total fumonisin contamination and their producing fungi in fresh and stored sorghum grain in east Haraghe, Ethiopia. Food Additives and Contaminants: Part B. 2016;**9**(4):237-245

[66] Mahammed A, Chala A, Dejene M, Finisia C, Hoisington DA, Sobolev VS, et al. Aspegillus and aflatoxin in groundnut (*Arachis hypogaea* L.) and groundnut cake in eastern Ethiopia. Food Additives and Contaminants: Part B. 2016;**9**(4):290-298

[67] Kollia E, Tsourflis K, Markaki P. Aflatoxin b1 in sesame seeds and sesame production from the Greek market. Food Additives and Contaminants: Part B. 2016;**9**(3):217-222

[68] Agbetiameh D, Ortega-Beltran A, Awuah R, Atehnkeng J, Cooty P, Bandopadhyay R. Prevalence of aflatoxin contamination in maize and groundnut in Ghana: Population structure, distribution, and toxigenicity of casual agents. Plant Disease. 2018;**102**(4):764-772

[69] Jayashree M, Wesley E. Effect of moisture content on aflatoxin production in field infected and farmer saved sorghum (FSS) grains. The International Journal of Analytical and Experimental Modal Analysis. 2019;**11**(11):2506

[70] Mukherjee A, Sharma M, Latkar SS. A study on aflatoxin content in black scented rice in India. International Journal of Pharmacy and Analytical Research. 2019;**8**(1):125-130

[71] Eslami M, Mashak Z, Heshmati A, Shokrzadeh M, Mozaffari Nejad AS. Determination of aflatoxin B1 levels in Iranian rice by ELISA method. Toxin Reviews. 2015;**34**(3):125-128

[72] Camardo Leggieri M, Bertuzzi T, Pietri A, Battilani P. Mycotoxin occurrence in maize produced in Northern Italy over the years 2009-2011: Focus on the role of crop related factors. Phytopathologica Mediterranea. 2015;**54**:212-221

[73] Kange AM, Cheruiyot EK, Ogendo JO, Arama PF. Effect of Sorghum (*Sorghum bicolor* L. Moench) grain conditions on occurrence of mycotoxin-producing fungi. Agriculture and food. Security. 2015;**4**(1):15

[74] Nafula SN, Misihairabgwi JM, Block R, Ishola A, Sulyok M, Krska R. Variation of fungal metabolites in sorghum malts used to prepare Namibian traditional fermented beverages Omaloduand Otombo. Toxins. 2019;**11**(3):165

[75] Apen D, Ochai D, Adejumo A, Muhammad H, Saidu A, Atehnkeng J, et al. Mycotoxicological concerns with sorghum,millet and seame in Northern Nigeria. Journal of Analytical Bioanalytical Techniques. 2016;**7**:336

[76] Rofiat AS, Fanelli F, Atanda O, Sulyok M, Cozzi G, Bavaro S, et al. Fungal and bacterial metabolites associated with natural contamination of locally processed rice (*Oryza sativa* L.) in Nigeria. Food Additives and Contaminants: Part A. 2015;**32**(6):950-959

[77] Asghar MA, Iqbal J, Ahmad A, Shamsuddin Z, Khan M. Incidence of

aflatoxins in export quality basmati rice collected from different areas of Pakistan. Science, Technology and Development (Pakistan). 2016;**32**(2):110-119

[78] Coloma Z, Oliveira M, Dilkin P, Mallmann A, Almeida C, Mallmann C. Mycotoxin occurrence in Peruvian purple maize. World Mycotoxin Journal. 2019;**12**(3):307-315

[79] Torovic L. Aflatoxins and ochratoxin A in flour: A survey of the Serbian retail market. Food Additives and Contaminants: Part B. 2018;**11**(1):26-32

[80] Kim DH, Hong SY, Kang JW, Cho SM, Lee KR, An TK, et al. Simultaneous determination of multi-mycotoxins in cereal grains collected from South Korea by LC/MS/MS. Toxins. 2017;**9**(3):106

[81] Lien KW, Wang X, Pan MH, Ling MP. Assessing aflatoxin exposure risk from peanuts and peanut products imported to Taiwan. Toxins. 2019;**11**(2):80

[82] Artic N, Konar N, Ozkan M, Cakmakci ML. Aflatoxin and genetically modified organisms analysis in Turkish corn. Food and Nutrition Sciences. 2016;**7**(2):138-148

[83] Turksoy S, Kabak B. Determination of aflatoxins and ochratoxin A in wheat from different regions of Turkey by HPLC with fluorescence detection. Acta Alimentaria. 2020;**49**(1):118-124

[84] Lavkor I, Var I, Saglam S, Uckun O, Tekin A, Savas O. Presence of some mycotoxins in peanuts from harvest to storage. Legume Research—An International Journal. 2019;**42**(6):862-866

[85] Newberne PM. Mycotoxins: Toxicity, carcinogenicity and the influence of various nutritional conditions. Environmental Health Perspectives. 1974;**9**:1-32

[86] Cavalheiro ACL. Aflatoxins and aflatoxicosis a review. World's Poultry Science Journal. 1981;**37**:34-38

[87] Malkinson M, Shlosberg A, Egyed MN, Avidar Y, Perl S, Weisman Y, et al. Hepatic cirrhosis suggesting aflatoxicosis in a flock of geese. Veterinary Record. 1982;**110**:101-103

[88] Leeson S, Diaz GJ, Summers JD. Aflatoxins. In: Poultry Metabolic Disorders and Mycotoxins. Guelph, Canada: University Books; 1995

[89] Diaz GJ, Sugahara M. Individual and combined effects of aflatoxin and gizzerosine in broiler chickens. British Poultry Science. 1995;**36**:729-736

[90] Diaz GJ, Calabrese E, Blain R. Aflatoxicosis in chickens (*Gallus gallus*): An example of hormesis? Poultry Science. 2008;**87**(4):727-732

[91] Muller RD, Carlson CW, Semeniuk G, Harshfield GS. The response of chicks, ducklings, goslings, pheasants and poults to graded levels of aflatoxins. Poultry Science. 1970;**49**(5):1346-1350

[92] Jones FT, Beth M, Genter MM, Hagler WM, Hansen JA, Mowrewy BA, et al. Understanding and Coping with Effects of Mycotoxins in Livestock Feed and Forage. Electronic publication No. DRO-29. Raleigh, North Carolina: NCCES, North Carolina State Univ.; 1994

[93] Asplin FD, Carnaghan RBA. The toxicity of certain groundnut meals for poultry with special reference to their effect on ducklings and chickens. Veterinary Record. 1961;**73**:1215-1219

[94] Mishra SK, Jena CR, Naik PK, Kumar D, Swain BK, Panda SK, et al. Impact of dietary aflatoxin-B1 on juvenile growth in white Pekin ducks. Indian Journal of Animal Research. 2022;**56**:175-181

[95] ASR. Annual Scientific Report. ICAR-Directorate on Poultry Research, Hyderabad, India, Published. Hyderabad, India: ICAR-DPR; 2021

[96] Mishra SK. Evidence of genetic-background impacting duck's susceptibility to Aflatoxicosis more than climate in terms of mortality and productivity-drops in tropical Indian conditions. In: S12-0053, Proceedings, XXV World's Poultry Congress, September 5-9, 2016, Beijing. China: World's Poultry Science Association (WPSA), WPSA-China and Chinese association of Animal Sciences and Veterinary medicine (CCAAV). 2016

[97] Hetzel DJS, Hoffmann D, Van De Ven J, Soeripto S. Mortality rate and liver histopathology in four breeds of ducks following long term exposure to low levels of aflatoxins. Singapore Veterinary Journal. 1984;**8**:6-14

[98] Calnek BC, Barnes HJ, McDougald LR, Saif YM. Diseases of Poultry. 10th ed. Ames, Iowa, USA: Mosby-Wolfe, Iowa State Univ. Press; 1997. pp. 951-979

[99] Chen X, Horn N, Applegate TJ. Efficiency of hydrated sodium calcium aluminosilicate to ameliorate the adverse effects of graded levels of aflatoxin B1 in broiler chicks. Poultry Science. 2014;**93**:2037-2047

[100] Fin CD, Mallmann CA, Dilkin P, Giacomini LZ, Machado LV, Mallmann AL. Effects of aflatoxins on the performance of pekin ducklings. Proceedings, XXIV World's Poultry Congress, Salvador—Bahia—Brazil. World's Poultry Science Association; 5-9 August 2012

[101] Ali I, Panda SK, Pati S, Acharya AP, Mishra SK, Jena GR, et al. Patho- morphological and genotoxic changes in induced aflatoxicosis in white Pekin ducks (Anas platyrhynchos domesticus). International Journal of Current Microbiology and Applied Sciences. 2019;**8**(05):1225-1233

[102] Gumbmann MR, Williams SN, Booth AN, Vohra P, Ernst RA, Bethard M. Aflatoxin susceptibility in various breeds of oultry. Proceedings of the Society for Experimental Biology and Medicine. 1970;**134**(3):683-688

[103] Arafa AS, Bloomer RJ, Wilson HR, Simpson CF, Harms RH. Susceptibility of various poultry species to dietary aflatoxin. British Poultry Science. 1981;**22**:431-436

[104] Lozano MC, Diaz GJ. Microsomal and cytosolic biotransformation of aflatoxin B1 in four poultry species. British Poultry Science. 2006;**47**:734-741

[105] Rawal S, Kim JE, Coulombe R. Aflatoxin B1 in poultry: Toxicology, metabolism and prevention. Research in Veterinary Science. 2010;**89**:325-331

[106] Yip SS, Coulombe RA. Molecular cloning and expression of a novel cytochrome P450 from Turkey liver with aflatoxin B1 oxidizing activity. Chemical Research in Toxicology. 2006;**19**:30-37

[107] Rawal S, Mendoza KM, Reed KM, Coulombe RA Jr. Structure, genetic mapping, and function of the cytochrome P450 3A37 gene in the Turkey (Meleagris gallopavo). Cytogenetics and Genome Research. 2009;**125**:67-73

[108] Rawal S, Coulombe RA Jr. Metabolism of aflatoxin B1 in Turkey liver microsomes: The relative roles of cytochromes P450 1A5 and 3A37. Toxicology and Applied Pharmacology. 2011;**254**:349-354

[109] Quist CF, Bounous DI, Kilburn JV, Nettles VF, Wyatt RD. The effect of dietary aflatoxin on wild Turkey poults. Journal of Wildlife Diseases. 2000;**36**:436-444

[110] Pandey I, Chauhan SS. Studies on production performance and toxin residues in tissues and eggs of layer chickens fed on diets with various concentrations of aflatoxin AFB1. British Poultry Science. 2007;**48**:713-723

[111] Giambrone JJ, Diener UL, Davis ND, Panangala VS, Hoerr FJ. Effects of aflatoxin on young turkeys and broiler chickens. Poultry Science. 1985;**64**:1678-1684

[112] Quezada T, Cuéllar H, Jaramillo-Juárez F, Valdivia AG, Reyes JL. Effects of aflatoxin B1 on the liver and kidney of broiler chickens during development. Comparative Biochemistry and Physiology Part C: Toxicology and Pharmacology. 2000;**125**:265-272

[113] Lee JT, Jessen KA, Beltran R, Starkl V, Schatzmayr G, Borutova R, et al. Mycotoxin-contaminated diets and deactivating compound in laying hens: 1. Effects on performance characteristics and relative organ weight. Poultry Science. 2012;**91**:2089-2095

[114] Hamilton PB, Tung HS, Harris JR, Gainer JH, Donaldson WE. The effect of dietary fat on aflatoxicosis in turkeys. Poultry Science. 1972;**51**:165-170

[115] Siller WG, Ostler DC. The histopathology of an entero hepatic system of Turkey poults. Veterinary Record. 1961;**73**:134

[116] Wannop CC. The histopathology of Turkey "X" disease in Great Britain. Avian Diseases. 1961;**5**:371-381

[117] Richard JL, Stubblefield RD, Lyon RL, Peden WM, Thurston JR, Rimler RB. Distribution and clearance of aflatoxins B1 and M1 in turkeys fed diets containing 50 or 150 ppb aflatoxin from naturally contaminated corn. Avian Diseases. 1986;**30**:788-793

[118] Monson MS, Coulombe RA, Reed KM. Aflatoxicosis: Lessons from toxicity and responses to aflatoxin B1 in poultry. Agriculture. 2015;**5**:742-777. DOI: 10.3390/agriculture5030742

[119] Sawhney DS, Vadehra DV, Baker RC. Aflatoxicosis in the laying Japanese quail. Poultry Science. 1973;**52**:485-493

[120] Sawhney DS, Vadehra DV, Baker RC. The metabolism of 14C aflatoxins in laying hens. Poultry Science. 1973;**52**:1302-1309

[121] Dhanasekaran D, Panneerselvam A, Thajuddin N. Evaluation of aflatoxicosis inhens fed with commercial poultry feed. Turkish Journal of Veterinary and Animal Sciences. 2009;**33**(5):385-391

[122] Jayabarathi P, Mohamudha P. Biochemical and histopathological analysis of aflatoxicosis in growing hens fed with commercial poultry feed. International Journal of Pharmaceutical Sciences Review and Research. 2010;**3**(2):127-130

[123] Azzam AH, Gabal MA. Aflatoxin and immunity in layer hens. Avian Pathology. 1998;**27**:570-577

[124] Oliveira CA, Rosmaninho JF, Butkeraitis P, Corrêa B, Reis TA, Guerra JL, et al. Effect of low levels of dietary aflatoxin B1 on laying Japanese quail. Poultry Science. 2002;**81**:976-980

[125] Olievera CF, Rosmaninho JF, Castro AL, Butkeraitis P, Reis TA, Correa B. Aflatoxin residues in eggs of laying Japanese quails after long term administration of rations containing low

levels of aflatoxin B1. Food Additives Contaminants. 2003;**20**:648-653

[126] Khan WA, Khan MZ, Khan A, Hassan ZU, Rafique S, Saleemi MK, et al. Dietary vitamin E in white leghorn layer breeder hens: A strategy to combat aflatoxin B1-induced damage. Avian Pathology. 2014;**43**:389-395

[127] Refai MK, Elbatrawi A, Osman G, Hassan A. Monograph on Avian Mycoses & Mycotoxicoses, A guide for Postgraduate Students. Giza, Egypt: Cairo University; 2016. Available from: https://www.academia.edu.eg./7688721-AtefHassan. https://www.researchgate.net/publication/Atef Hassan

[128] Bertuzzi T, Rastelli S, Mulazzi A, Pietri A. Evaluation and improvement of extraction methods for the analysis of aflatoxins B1, B2, G1 and G2 from naturally contaminated maize. Food Analytical Methods. 2012;**5**(3):512-519

[129] Taylor SL, King JW, Richard JL, Greer JI. Analytical scale supercritical fluid extraction of aflatoxin B1 from field inoculated corn. Journal of Agricultural and Food Chemistry. 1993;**41**(6):910-913

[130] Stroka J, Petz M, Joerissen U, Anklam E. Investigation of various extractants for the analysis of aflatoxin B1 in different food and feed matrices. Feed Additives and Contaminants. 1999;**16**(8):331-338

[131] Lee NA, Wang S, Allan RD, Kennedy IR. A rapid aflatoxin B1 Elisa: Development and validation with reduced matrix effects for peanuts, corn, pistachio, and soybeans. Journal of Agricultural and Food Chemistry. 2004;**52**(10):2746-2755

[132] Ma FJ, Chen R, Li P, Zhang Q, Zhang W, Hu X. Preparation of an immunoaffinity column with amino-silica gel microparticles and its application in sample cleanup for aflatoxin detection in agri-products. Molecules. 2013;**18**(2):2222-2235

[133] Shelver WL, Larsen GL, Huwe JK. Use of an immunoaffinity column for tetra chloro di benzo-p-dioxin serum sample clean up. Journal of Chromatography B: Biomedical Applications. 1998;**705**(2):261-268

[134] Kumar P, Mahato DK, Kamle M, Mohanta TK, Kang SG. Aflatoxins: A global concern for food safety, human health and their management. Frontier in Microbiology. 2017;**7**:2170

[135] Herzallah SM. Determination of aflatoxins in eggs, milk, meat and meat products using HPLC, fluorescent and UV detectors. Food Chemistry. 2009;**114**:1141-1146

[136] AlFaris NA, Wabaidur SM, Alothman ZA, Altamimi JZ, Aldayel TS. Fast afficient immunoaffinity column cleanup and liquid chromatography-tandem mass spectrometry method for the quantitative analysis of aflatoxins in baby food and feeds. Journal of Separation Science. 2020;**9**:644

[137] Carvalho K, Goncalves G, Lopes A, Santos E, Vargas E, Magalhaes W. Modelling uncertainty estimation for the determination of aflatoxin M1 in milk by visual and densitometric thin-layer chromatography with immunoaffinity column cleanup. Food Additives and Contaminants Part A. 2012;**29**:679-693

[138] Asadi M. Separation and quantification of aflatoxin in grains using modified dispersive liquid-liquid microextraction combined with high performance liquid chromatography. Journal of Food Measurement and Characterization. 2020;**14**:925-930

[139] Musundire R, Osuga IM, Cheseto X, Irungu J, Torto B. Aflatoxin

contamination detected in nutrient and anti-oxidant rich edible stink bug stored in recycled grain containers. PLoS One. 2016;**11**:1-6

[140] Sulyok M, Beed F, Boni S, Abbas A, Mukunzi A, Krska R. Quantitation of multiple mycotoxins and cyanogenic glucosides in cassava samples from Tanzania and Rwanda by an LC-MS/MS based multi-toxin method. Food Additives and Contaminants Part A. 2015;**32**:488-502

[141] Stroka J, Anklam E. New strategies for the screening and determination of aflatoxin and the detection of aflatoxin-producing moulds in food and feed. TrAc-Trends in Analytical Chemistry. 2002;**21**(2):90-95

[142] Paap E, H-Otta K, Zaray G, Minscovics E. Liquid chromatographic determination of aflatoxins. Microchemical Journal. 2002;**73**(1-2):39-46

[143] Nawaz S, Coker RD, Haswell SJ. Development and evaluation of analytical methodology for the determination of aflatoxins in palm kernels. The Analyst. 1992;**117**(1):67-74

[144] Ramesh J, Sarathchandra G, Sureshkumar V. Analysis of feed samples for aflatoxin B1 contamination by HPTLC-a validated method. International Journal of Current Microbiology and Applied Sciences. 2013;**2**:373-377

[145] Tao F, Yao H, Hruska Z, Burger LW, Rajasekaran K, Bhatnagar D. Recent development of optical methods in rapid and non-destructive detection of aflatoxin and fungal contamination in agricultural products. Trends in Analytical Chemistry. 2018;**100**:65-81

[146] Hussain A, Afzal A, Irfan M, Malik KA. Molecular detection of aflatoxin producing strains of *aspergillus flavus* from peanut (*Arachis hypogaea*). Turkish Journal of Agriculture, Food Science and Technology. 2015;**3**:335-341

[147] Yang ZY, Shim WB, Kim JH, Park SJ, Kang SJ, Nam BS, et al. Detection of aflatoxin-producing molds in Korean fermented foods and grains by multiplex PCR. Journal of Food Protection. 2004;**67**(11):2622-2626. DOI: 10.4315/0362-028x-67.11.2622

[148] Kim NY, Lee JH, Lee I, Ji GE. An evaluation of aflatoxin and cyclopiazonic acid production in aspergillus oryzae. Journal of Food Protection. 2014;**77**:1010-1016

[149] Wu D, Sun DW. Advanced application of hyperspectral imaging technology for food quality and safety analysis and assessment: A review-part 1:Fundamentals. Innovative Food Science and Emerging Technologies. 2013;**19**:1-14

[150] Ropodi AI, Panagou EZ, Nychas GJE. Data mining derived from food analyses using non-invasive/non-destructive analytical techniques; determination of food authenticity, quality & safety in tandem with computer science discipline. Trends in Food Science and Technology. 2016;**50**:11-25

[151] Shrestha S, Knapie M, Zibrat U, Deleuran LC, Gislum R. Single seed near-infrared hyperspectral imaging in determining tomato (*Solanum lycopersicum* L.) seed quality in association with multivariate data analysis. Sensors and Actuators B: Chemical. 2016;**237**:1027-1034

[152] Siche R, Vejarano R, Aredo V, Velasquez L, Saldana E, Quevedo R. Evaluation of food quality and safety with hyperspectral imaging (HSI). Food Engineering Review. 2016;**8**:306-322

[153] Pearson TC, Wicklow DT. Detection of corn kernels infected by fungi. Transactions of American Society of

Agricultural and Biological Engineers. 2006;**49**:1235-1245

[154] Williams PJ, Geladi P, Britz TJ, Manley M. Investigation of fungal development in maize kernels using NIR hyperspectral imaging and multivariate data analysis. Journal of Cereal Science. 2012;**55**:272-278

[155] Wang W, Heitschmidt GW, Windham WR, Feldner P, Ni X, Chu X. Feasibility of detecting aflatoxin B1 on inoculated maize kernels surface using Vis/NIR hyperspectral imaging. Journal of Food Science. 2015;**80**:M116-M122

[156] Wang W, Ni X, Lawrence KC, Yoon SC, Heitschmidt GW, Feldner P. Feasibility of detecting aflatoxin B1 in single maize kernels using hyperspectral imaging. Journal of Food Engineering. 2015;**166**:182-192

[157] Saeger SD, Sibanda L, Peteghem CV. Analysis of zearalenone and zearalenol in animal feed using high-performance liquid chromatography. Analytica Chemica Acta. 2003;**487**:137-143

[158] Berthiller F, Schuhmacher R, Buttinger G, Krska R. Rapid simultaneous determination of major type-A- and B-trichothecenes as well as zearalenone in maize by high performance liquid chromatography-tandem mass spectrometry. Journal of Chromatography A. 2005;**1062**:209-216

[159] Zollner P, Mayer-Helm B. Trace mycotoxin analysis in complex biological and food matrices by liquid chromatography-atmospheric pressure ionization mass spectrometry. Journal of Chromatography A. 2006;**1136**:123-169

[160] Njobeh PP, Dutton MF, Aberg AT, Haggblom P. Estimation of multi-mycotoxin contamination in south African compound feed. Toxins. 2012;**4**:836-848

[161] Waskiewicz A, Beszterda M, Golinski P. Occurrence of fumonisins in food—An interdisciplinary approach to the problem. Food Control. 2012;**26**:491-499

[162] Seo DG, Phat C, Kim DH, Lee C. Occurrence of fusarium mycotoxin Fumonosin B1 and B2 in animal feeds in Korea. Mycotoxin Research. 2013;**29**:159-167

[163] Trucksess MW, Diaz-Amigo C. Mycotoxin in foods. In: Nriagu JO, editor. Reference Modules in Earth Systems and Environmental Sciences, Encyclopedia of Environment Health. Burlington, MA, USA: Elsevier; 2011. pp. 888-897

[164] Fung F, Clark RF. Health effects of mycotoxins: A toxicological overview. Journal of Toxicology-Clinical Toxicology. 2004;**42**:217-234

[165] Zheng MZ, Richard JL, Binder J. A review of rapid methods for the analysis of mycotoxins. Mycopathologica. 2006;**161**:261-273

[166] Berthiller F, Sulyok M, Krska R, Schuhmacher R. Chromatographic methods for the simultaneous determination of mycotoxins and their conjugates in cereals. International Journal of Food Microbiology. 2007;**119**:33-37

[167] Mahfuz M, Gazi MA, Hossain M, Islam MR, Fahim SM, Ahmad T. General and advanced methods for the detection and measurement of aflatoxins and aflatoxin metabolites: A review. Toxin Reviews. 2018;**39**(2):123-137

[168] Ouakhssase A, Chahid A, Choubbane H, Aitmazirt A, Addi EA. Optimization and validation of a liquid chromatography/tandem mass spectrometry (LC-MS/MS) method for the determination of aflatoxins in maize. Heliyon. 2019;**5**(5):e01565

[169] Rathod RH, Chaudhuri SR, Patil AS, Shirkhedhar A. Ultra-high performance liquid chromatography-MS/MS (UHPLC-MS/MS) in practice. Analysis of drugs and pharmaceutical formulations. Future Journal of Pharmaceutical Sciences. 2019;**59**(1):6

[170] Pal A, Acharya D, Saha D, Dhar TK. Development of a membrane-based immune filtration assay for the detection of T-2 toxin. Analytical Chemistry. 2004;**76**(14):4237-4240

[171] Matabaro E, Ishimwe N, Uwimbabazi E, Lee BH. Current immunoassay methods for the rapid detection of aflatoxin in milk and dairy products. Comprehensive Reviews in Food Science and Food Safety. 2017;**16**(5):808-820

[172] Durmus E, Gunes A, Kalkan H. Detection of aflatoxin and surface mould contaminated figs by using Fourier transform near-infrared reflectance spectroscopy. Journal of the Science of Food and Agriculture. 2017;**97**(1):317-323

[173] Alcaide-Molina M, Ruiz-Jimenez J, Mata-Granados J, de Castro ML. High through-put aflatoxin determination in plant material by automated solid-phase extraction on-line coupled to laser-induced fluorescence screening and determination by liquid chromatography-triple quadrupole mass spectrometry. Journal of Chromatography A. 2009;**1216**(7):1115-1125

[174] Gloria EMD, Fonseca H, Calori-Domingues MA, Souza I. Evaluation of the black light test for screening aflatoxin contaminated maize in the Brazilian food industry. Food Additives and Contaminats. 1998;**15**(2):181-184

[175] Sheibani A, Tabrizchi M, Ghaziaskar HS. Determination of aflatoxin B1 and B2 using ion mobility spectrometry. Talanta. 2008;**75**(1):233-238

[176] Matumba L, Poucke V, Ediage EN, Jacobs B, De Saeger S. Effectiveness of hand sorting, flotation/washing, dehulling and combinations thereof on the decontamination of mycotoxin-contaminated white maize. Food Additives and Contaminants Part A. 2015;**32**:960-969

[177] Peng Z, Chen L, Zhu Y, Huang Y, Hu X, Wu Q, et al. Current major degradation methods for aflatoxins: A review. Trends in Food Science and Technology. 2018;**80**:155-166

[178] Siwela AH, Siwela M, Matindi G, Dube S, Nziramasanga N. Decontamination of aflatoxin-contaminated maize by dehulling. Journal of the Science of Food and Agriculture. 2005;**85**:2535-2538

[179] Fandohan P, Zoumenou D, Hounhouigan DJ, Marasas WFO, Wingfield MJ, Hell K. Fate of aflatoxins and fumonisins during the processing of maize into food products in Benin. International Journal of Food Microbiology. 2005;**98**:249-259

[180] Mutungi C, Lamuka P, Arimi S, Gathumbi J, Onyango C. The fate of aflatoxin during processing of maize into muthukoi—A traditional Kenyan food. Food Control. 2008;**19**:714-721

[181] Castells M, Ramos AJ, Sanchis V, Marin S. Distribution of total aflatoxins in milled fraction of dehulled rice. Journal of Agriculture and Food Chemistry. 2007;**55**:2760-2764

[182] Panda AK. Mycotoxicosis: Its prevention and control. In: Recent Advances in Broiler Chicken Nutrition. 1st ed. Hyderabad, India: Hind Publications; 2014. p. p459

[183] Jones F. Controlling mould growth in feeds. Feed International. 1987;**8**:20-26

[184] Herzallah S, Alshawabkeh K, Fataftah AAL. Aflatoxin decontamination of artificially contaminated feeds by sunlight, ϒ-radiation, and microwave heating. Journal of Applied Poultry Research. 2008;**17**:515-521

[185] Arzandeh S, Jinap S. Effect of initial aflatoxin concentration, heating time and roasting temperature on aflatoxin reduction in contaminated peanuts and process optimization using response surface modeling. International Journal of Food Science and Technology. 2011;**46**:485-491

[186] Hwang JH, lee KG. Reduction of aflatoxin B1 contamination in wheat by various cooking treatments. Food Chemistry. 2006;**98**:71-75

[187] Raters M, Matissek R. Thermal stability of aflatoxin B1 and ochratoxin A. Mycotoxin Research. 2008;**24**:130-134

[188] Lee J, Her JY, Lee KG. Reduction of aflatoxins (B1, B2, G1, G2) in soybean-based model systems. Food Chemistry. 2015;**189**:45-51

[189] Perez-FloresGC,Moreno-MartinezE, Mendez-Albores A. Effect of microwave heating during alkaline-cooking of aflatoxin contaminated maize. Journal of Food Science. 2011;**76**(2):T48-T52

[190] Di Stefano V, Pitonzo R, Avellone G. Effect of gamma irradiation on aflatoxins and ochratoxin A reduction in almond samples. Journal of Food Research. 2014;**3**:113

[191] Di Stefano V, Pitonzo R, Cicero N, D'Oca MC. Mycotoxin contamination of animal feeding stuff: Detoxification by gamma-irradiation and reduction of aflatoxins and ochratoxin A concentrations. Food Additives and Contaminants Part A. 2014;**31**:2034-2039. DOI: 10.1080/19440049.2014.968882

[192] Iqbal SZ, Bhatti IA, Asi MR, Zuber M, Shahid M, Parveen I. Effect of ϒ-irradiation on fungal load and aflatoxins reduction in red chillies. Radiation Physics and Chemistry. 2013;**82**:80-84

[193] Jalili M, Jinap S, Noranizan MA. Aflatoxin and ochratoxin A reduction in black and white pepper by gamma radiation. Radiation Physics and Chemistry. 2012;**81**:1786-1788

[194] Mohamad NF, El-dine RSS, Aly M, Kotb M, Saber A. Assessing the possible effect of gamma irradiation on the reduction of aflatoxin B1, and on the moisture content in some cereal grains. American Journal of Biomedical Science. 2015;**7**:33-39

[195] Rushing BR, Selim MI. Effect of dietary acids on formation of aflatoxin B2a as a means to detoxify aflatoxin B1. Food Additives contamination Part A Chemical Analytical control Exposure risk Assess. 2016;**33**:1456-1467

[196] Safara M, Zaini F, Hashemi SJ, Mahmoudi M, Khosravi AR, Shojai-Aliabadi F. Aflatoxin detoxification in rice using citric acid. Iranian Journal of Public Health. 2010;**39**:24-29

[197] Mendez-Albores A, Del Rio-Garcia JC, Moreno-Martinez E. Decontamination of aflatoxin duckling feed with aqueous citric acid treatment. Animal Feed Science and Technology. 2007;**135**:249-262

[198] Mendez-Albores A, Martinez-Bustos F, Gaytan-Martinez M, Moreno-Martinez E. Effect of lactic and citric acid on the stability of B-aflatoxins in extrusion cooked sorghum. Letters in Applied Microbiology. 2008;**47**:1-7

[199] Bagley EB. Decontamination of corn containing aflatoxin by treatment with ammonia. Journal of American Oil Chemist's Society. 1979;**56**:808-811

[200] Galılı A, Naguib K. Effect of high pressure ammoniation procedure on the detoxification of aflatoxins parasiticus which was used to contaminate the yellow corn. Mycotoxin Research. 1997;**13**:23-34

[201] Weng CY, Park DL, Martinez AJ. Efficacy and permanency of ammonia treatment in reducing aflatoxin levels in corn. Food Additives and Contaminants. 1994;**11**:649-658

[202] Rushing BR, Selim MI. Aflatoxin B1: A review on metabolism, toxicity, occurrence in food, occupational exposure, and detoxification methods. Food and Chemical Toxicology. 2019;**124**:81-100

[203] Isikber AA, Athanassiou CG. The use of ozone gas for the control of insects and micro-organisms in stored products. Journal of Stored Products Research. 2015;**64**:139-145

[204] El-Desouky T, Sharoba A, El-Desouky A, El-Mansy H, Naguib K. Effect of ozone gas on degradation of aflatoxin B1 and aspergillus flavus fungi. Journal of Environmental and Analytical Toxicology. 2012;**2**:1-6

[205] Chen R, Ma F, Li PW, Zhang W, Ding XX, Zhang Q, et al. Effects of ozone on aflatoxins detoxification and nutritional quality of peanuts. Food Chemistry. 2014;**146**:284-288

[206] de Alencar ER, Faroni LRDA, Soares N d FF, da Silva WA, da Silva Carvallho MC. Efficacy of ozone as a fungicidal and detoxifying agent of aflatoxins in peanuts. Journal of The Science of Food and Agriculture. 2012;**92**:899-905

[207] Diao E, Hou H, Chen B, Shan C, Dong H. Ozonolysis efficiency and safety evaluation of aflatoxinB1 in peanuts. Food and Chemical Toxicology. 2013;**5**:519-525

[208] Inan F, Pala M, Doymaz I. Use of ozone in detoxification of aflatoxin B1 in red pepper. Journal of Stored Products Research. 2007;**43**:425-429

[209] Luo X, Wang R, Wang L, Li Y, Bian Y, Chen Z. Effect of ozone treatment on aflatoxin B1 and safety evaluation of ozonised corn. Food Control. 2014;**37**:171-176

[210] Luo X, Wang R, Wang L, Li Y, Wang Y, Chen Z. Detoxification of aflatoxin in corn flour by ozone. Journal of The Science of Food and Agriculture. 2014;**94**:2253-2258

[211] Torlak E, Akata I, Erci F, Uncu AT. Use of gaseous ozone to reduce aflatoxin B1 and microorganisms in poultry feed. Journal of Stored Product Research. 2016;**68**:44-49

[212] Ismail A, Goncalves BL, de Neeff DV, Ponzilacqua B, Cppa CFSC, Hintzsche H, et al. Aflatoxin in foodstuffs: Occurrence and recent advances in decontamination. Food Research International. 2018;**113**:74-85

[213] Loi M, Renaud JB, Rosini E, Pollegioni L, Vignali E, Haidukowski M, et al. Enzymatic transformation of aflatoxin B1 by Rh_DypB peroxidase and characterization of reaction products. Chemosphere. 2020;**250**:12696

[214] El-Nezami H, Kankaanpaa P, Salminen S, Ahokas J. Ability of dairy strain of lactic acid bacteria to bind a common food carcinogen, aflatoxin B1. Food and Chemical Toxicology. 1998;**36**:321-326

[215] El-Nezami H, Mykkanen H, Kankaanpaa P, Salminen S, Ahokas J. Ability of Lactobacillus

and Propionibacterium strains to remove aflatoxin B1 from the chicken duodenum. Journal of Food Protection. 2000;**63**(4):549-552

[216] Brana MT, Cimmarusti MT, Haidukowski M, Logrieco AF, Altomare C. Bioremediation of aflatoxin B1 contaminated maize by king oyster mushroom (*Pleurotuseryngii*). PlosOne. 2017;**12**:1-14

[217] Farzaneh M, Shi ZQ, Ghassempour A, Sedaghat N, Ahmadzadeh M, Mirabolfathy M, et al. Aflatoxin B1 degradationby Bacillus subtilis UTBSP1 isolated from pistachio nuts of Iran. Food Control. 2012;**23**:100-106

[218] Hamad GM, Taha TH, Hafez EE, Ali SH, El-Sohaimy SA. Supplementation of Cerelac baby food with yeast probiotic cocktail strains induces high potential for aflatoxin detoxification both *in vitro* and *in vivo* in mother and baby albino rats. Journal of the Science of Food and Agriculture. 2017;**98**:707-718

[219] Haskard CA, El-Nezami HS, Kankaanpaa PE, Salminen S, Ahokas JT. Surface binding of aflatoxin B1 by lactic acid bacteria. Applied Environmental Microbiology. 2001;**67**:3086-3091

[220] Liu J, Song WJ, Zhang NY, Tan J, Kumar CS, Sun LH, et al. Biodetoxification of aflatoxin B1 in cottonseed meal by fermentation of Cellulosimicrobiumfunkei in duckling diet. Poultry Science. 2017;**96**:923-930

[221] Oluwafemi F, Kumar M, Bandyopadhyay R, Ogunbanwo T, Ayanwande KB. Bio-detoxification of aflatoxin B1 in artificially contaminated maize grains using lactic acid bacteria. Toxin Reviews. 2010;**29**:115-122

[222] Pizzolitto RP, Armado MR, Salvano MA, Dalcero AM, Rosa CA. Evaluation of *Saccharomyces cerevisiae* as an antiaflatoxicogenic agent in broiler feedstuffs. Poultry Science. 2013;**92**(6):1655-1663

[223] Kusumaningtyas E, Widiastuti R, Myryam R. Reduction of aflatoxin B1 in chicken feed by using *Saccharomyces cerevisiae*, *Rhizopus oligosporus* and their combination. Mycopathologica. 2006;**162**(4):307-311

[224] Iram W, Anjum T, Iqbal M, Ghaffar A, Abbas M. Structural elucidation and toxicity assessment of degraded products of aflatoxin B1 and B2 by aqueous extracts of Trachyspermumammi. Frontier in Micrbiology. 2016;**7**(346):1-16. DOI: 10.3389/fmicb.2016.00346

[225] Iram W, Anjum T, Iqbal M, Ghaffar A, Abbas M, Khan AM. Structural analysis and biological toxicity of aflatoxin B1 and B2 degradation products following detoxification by Ocimumbasillicum and Cassia fistula aqeous extracts. Frontier in Microbiology. 2016;**7**:1-18. DOI: 10.3389/fmicb.2016.01105

[226] Velazhahan R, Vijayanandraj S, Vijayasamundeeswari A, Paranidharan V, Samiayappan R, Iwamoto T, et al. Detoxification of aflatoxins by seed extracts of the medicinal plant, *Trachyspermumammi* (L) Sprague ex Turrill-structural analysis and biological toxicity of degradation product of aflatoxin G1. Food Control. 2010;**21**:719-725

[227] Vijayanandraj S, Brinda R, Kannan K, Adhithya R, Vinothini S, Senthil K, et al. Detoxification of aflatoxin B1 by an aqueous extract from leaves of *Adhatod avasica* Nees. Microbiology Research. 2014;**169**:294-300

[228] Alberts JF, Gelderblom WCA, Botha A, Van Zyl WH. Degradation

of aflatoxin B1 by fungal laccase enzymes. International Journal of Food Microbiology. 2009;**135**:47-52

[229] Loi M, Fanelli F, Zucca P, Liuzzi V, Quintieri L, Cimmarusti M, et al. Aflatoxin B1 and M1 degradation by Lac2 from Pleurotuspulmonarius and redox mediators. Toxins. 2016;**8**:245

[230] Xu L, Ahmad MFE, Sangare L, Zhao Y, Selvaraj JN, Xing F, et al. Novel aflatoxin-dgrading enzyme from bacillus shackletonii. Toxins. 2017;**9**:36

[231] Yehia RS. Aflatoxin detoxification by manganese peroxidase purified from *Pleurotusostreatus*. Brazilian Journal of Microbiology. 2014;**45**:127-133

[232] Wlison H, Douglas C, Harms R, Edds G. Reduction of aflatoxin effects on quail. Poultry Science. 1975;**54**(3):923-925

[233] Denil M, Celik K, Okan F. Effects of vitamin A supplementary in the feed to reduce toxic effects of aflatoxin B1 on Japanese quails (*Coturnic coturnix japonica*). International Journal of Poultry Science. 2003;**2**(2):174-177

[234] Oguz H. A review from experimental trials on detoxification of aflatoxin in poultry feed. Eurasian Journal of Veterinary Science. 2011;**27**(1):1-12

[235] Surai P. Selenium in poultry nutrition 2.Reproduction,egg and meat quality and practical applications. World's Poultry Science Journal. 2002;**58**(04):431-450

[236] Surai P, Fisinin V. Selenium in poultry breeder nutrition: An update. Animal Feed Science and Technology. 2014;**191**:1-15

[237] Liao S, Shi D, Clemons-Chevis CL, Guo S, Su R, Qiang P, et al. Protective role of selenium on hepatic mitochondrial antioxidant capacity in ducklings intoxicated with aflatoxin B1. Biological Trace Element Research. 2014;**145**(3):325-329

[238] He Y, Fang J, Peng X, Cui H, Zuo Z, Deng J, et al. Effects of sodium selenite on aflatoxin B1-induced decrease of ileac T cell and the mRNA contents of IL-2,IL-6, and TNF-α in broilers. Biological Trace Element Research. 2014;**159**(1-3, 173):167

[239] Wang F, Shu G, Peng X, Fang J, Chen K, Cui H, et al. Protective effects of sodium selenite against aflatoxin B1-induced oxidative stress and apoptosis in broiler spleen. International Journal of Environmental Research and Public Health. 2013;**10**(7):2834-2844

[240] Peng X, Zhang S, Fang J, Cui H, Zuo Z, Deng J. Protective roles of sodium selenite against aflatoxin B1-induced apoptosis of jejunum in broilers. International Journal of Environmental Research and Public Health. 2014;**11**(12):13130-13143

[241] Peng X, Yu Z, Liang N, Chi X, Li X, Jiang M, et al. The mitochondrial and death receptor pathways involved in the thymocytes apoptosis induced by aflatoxin B1. Oncotarget. 2016;**7**(11):12222-12234

[242] Sun LH, Zhang NY, Zhu MK, Zhao L, Zhou JC, Qi DS. Prevention of aflatoxin B1 hepatoxicity by dietary selenium is associated with inhibition of cytochrome P450 isozymes and up-regulation of 6 Seleno protein genes in Chick liver. Journal of Nutrition. 2016;**46**(4):655-661

[243] Prasad AS. Essential and Toxic Element: Trace Elements in Human Health and Disease. Amsterdam: Elsevier; 2013

[244] Mills CF. Zinc in Human Biology. New York: Springer Science and Business Media; 2013

[245] Ho E. Zinc deficiency, DNA damage and cancer risk. The Journal of Nutritional Biochemistry. 2004;**15**(10):572-578

[246] Hegazy S, Adachi Y. Comparison of the effects of dietary selenium, zinc, and selenium and zinc supplementation on growth and immune response between chick groups that were inoculated with Salmonella and aflatoxin or Salmonella. Poultry Science. 2000;**79**(3):331-335

[247] Powel SR. The antioxidant properties of zinc. Journal of Nutrition. 2000;**130**(5):1447S-1454S

[248] Prasad AS, Bao B, Beck FW, Kucuk O, Sarkar FH. Antioxidant effect of zinc in humans. Free Radical Biology and Medicine. 2004;**37**(8):1182-1190

[249] Mansour SA, Mossa ATH. Lipid peroxidation and oxidative stress in rat erythrocytes induced by chlorpyrifos and the protective effect of zinc. Pesticide Biochemistry and Physiology. 2009;**93**(1):34-39

[250] Chen T, Cui H, Cui Y, Bai C, Gong T, Peng X. Cell-cycle blockage associated with increased apoptotic cells in the thymus of chickens fed on diets high in fluorine. Human and Experimental Toxicology. 2011;**30**(7):685-692

[251] Edrington TS, Kubena LF, Harvey RB, Rottinghaus GE. Influence of super activated charcoal on the toxic effects of aflatoxin or T-2 toxin in growing broilers. Poultry Science. 1997;**76**:1205-1211

[252] Dalvi RR, Ademoyero AA. Toxic effects of aflatoxin B1 in chickens given feed contaminated with *Aspergillous flavus* and reduction of toxicity by activated charcoal and some chemical agents. Avian Disease. 1984;**28**:61-69

[253] Dalvi RR, McGown C. Experimental induction of chronic aflatoxicosis in chickens by purified aflatoxin B1 and its reversal by activated charcoal, pheno barbitol, and reduced glutathione. Poultry Science. 1984;**63**:485-491

[254] Kubena LF, Harvey RB, Phillips TD, Corrier DE, Huff WE. Diminution of aflatoxicosis in growing chickens by dietary addition of a hydrated sodium calcium aluminosilicate. Poultry Science. 1990;**69**:727-735

[255] Edrington TS, Sarr AB, Kubena LF, Harvey RB, Phillips TD. Effect of hydrated sodium calcium aluminosilicate (HSCAS), acidic HSCAS and activated charcoal, on the metabolic profile and toxicity of aflatoxin B1 in turkey poults. Toxicology Letter. 1996;**89**:115-122

[256] Jindal N, Mahipal SK, Mahajan NK. Toxicity of AFB1 in broiler chicks and its reduction by activated charcoal. Research in Veterinary Science. 1994;**56**:3740

[257] Raju MVLN, Devegowda G. Influence of esterified-glucomannan on performance and organ morphology, serum biochemistry and haematology in broilers exposed to individual and combined mycotoxicosis (aflatoxin, ochratoxin and T-2 toxin). British Poultry Science. 2000;**41**(5):640-650

[258] Aravind KL, Patil VS, Devegowda G, Umakantha B, Ganpule SP. Efficacy of esterified glucomannan to counteract mycotoxicosis in naturally contaminated feed on performance and serum biochemical and hematological parameters in broilers. Poultry Science. 2003;**82**(4):571-576

[259] Mgbeahuruike AC, Tochukwu EE, Christian OC, Shoyinka VC, Karlsson M, Nordkvist E. Detoxification of aflatoxin-contaminated poultry feed by 3 adsorbents, bentonite, activated charcoal, and fuller's earth. Journal of Applied Poultry Research. 2018;**27**:461-471

[260] Hedayati M, Manafi M, Yari M. Aflatoxicosis in broilers: Efficacy of a commercial mycotoxin Binder on performance and immunity parameters. International Journal of Ecosystem. 2014;**4**(4):176-183

[261] Silambarasan S, Singh R, Mandal AB. Efficacy of certain adsorbents on carcass traits and livability of broiler chickens fed aflatoxin B1 contaminated diets. Indian Journal of Poultry Science. 2015;**50**(1):113-117

[262] Kubena LF, Harvey RB, Phillips TD, Heidelbaugh ND. Novel approach to the preventive management of aflatoxins in poultry. In: Proc. United States Animal Health Association. Richmond, VA: Lewis Printing Co.; 1987. pp. 302-304

[263] Phillips TD, Kubena LF, Harvey RB, Taylor DS, Heidelbaugh ND. Hydrated sodium calcium alluminosilicate: A high affinity sorbent for aflatoxin. Poultry Science. 1988;**67**:243-247

[264] Pasha TNMU, Farooq MU, Khattak FM, Jabar MA, Khan AD. Effectiveness of sodium bentonite and two commercial products as aflatoxin absorbents in diets for broiler chickens. Animal Feed Science and Technology. 2007;**132**:103-110

[265] Gowda NKS, Ledoux DR, Rottinghaus GE, Bermudez AJ, Chen YC. Efficacy of turmeric (*Curcuma longa*) containing a known level of curcumin, and a hydrated sodium calcium aluminosilicate to ameliorate the adverse effects of aflatoxin in broiler chicks. Poultry Science. 2008;**87**:1125-1130

[266] Karaca H, Nas S. Combined effect of P^H and heat treatment on degradation of aflatoxins in dried figs. Journal of Food Processing and Preservation. 2009;**33**:329-339

[267] Aly SE, Hathout AS. Fate of aflatoxin B1 in contaminated corn gluten during acid hydrolysis. Journal of the Science of Food and Agriculture. 2011;**91**:421-427

[268] Aiko V, Edamana P, Mehta A. Decomposition and detoxification of aflatoxin B1 by lactic acid. Journal of the Science of Food and Agriculture. 2016;**96**:1959-1966

[269] Rastegar H, Shoeibi S, Yazdanpanah H, Amirahmadi M, Khaneghah AM, Campagnollo FB, et al. Removal of aflatoxin B1 by roasting with lemon juice and/or citric acid in contaminated pistachio nuts. Food Control. 2017;**71**:279-284

[270] Marks HL, Wyatt RD. Aflatoxin susceptibility of selected and control Japanese quail lines. British Poultry Science. 1980;**21**:29-36

[271] Marks HL, Wyatt RD. Genetic resistance to aflatoxin in Japanese quail. Science. 1979;**206**:1329-1330

[272] Lanza GM, Washburn KW, Wyatt RD, Marks HL. Genetic variations of physiological response to aflatoxin in Gallus domesticus. Theoretical Applied Genetics. 1982;**63**:207-212

[273] Lanza GM, Washburn KW, Wyatt RD, Marks HL. Effect of dietary aflatoxin concentration on the assessment of genetic variability of response in a random bred population of chickens. Genetics. 1983;**104**:121-131

[274] Wyatt RD, Marks HL, Manning RO. Selection for resistance to aflatoxin

in chickens. Poultry Science. 1987;**66**:1901-1904

[275] Dupont C, Armant DR, Brenner CA. Epigenetics: Definition, mechanisms and clinical perspective. Seminars in Reproductive Medicine. 2009;**27**(05):351-357

[276] Yang IV, Schwartz DA. Epigenetic mechanisms and the development of asthma. Journal of Allergy and Clinical Immunology. 2012;**130**:1243-1255

[277] Chappell G, Pogribny IP, Guyton KZ, Rusyn I. Epigenetic alterations induced by genotoxic occupational and environmental human chemical carcinogens: A systematic literature review. Reviews in Mutation Research. 2016;**768**:27-45

[278] Ehrlich M, Gama-Sosa MA, Huang LH, Midgett RM, Kuo KC, McCune RA, et al. Amount and distribution of 5-methylcytosine in human DNA from different types of tissues of cells. Nucleic Acid Research. 1982;**10**:2709-2721

[279] Bird A. DNA methylation patterns and epigenetic memory. Genes Development. 2002;**16**:6-21

[280] Hernandez-Vargas H, Castelino J, Silver MJ, Dominguez-Salas P, Cros MP, Durand G, et al. Exposure to aflatoxin B1 in utero is associated with DNA methylation in white blood cells of infants in the Gambia. International Journal of Epidemiology. 2015;**44**(4):1238-1248

[281] Hong L, Ahuja N. DNA methylation biomarkers of stool and blood for early detection of colon cancer. Genetic Testing and Molecular Biomarkers. 2013;**17**:401-406

[282] Renner M, Wolf T, Meyer H, Hartmann W, Penzel R, Ulrich A, et al. Integrative DNA methylation and gene expression analysis in high-grade soft tissue sarcomas. Genome Biology. 2013;**14**:137

[283] Son JW, Jeong KJ, Jean WS, Park SY, Jheon S, Cho HM, et al. Genome-wide combination profiling of DNA copy number and methylation for deciphering biomarkers in non-small cell lung cancer patients. Cancer Letters. 2011;**311**:29-37

[284] Bondurant AE, Huang Z, Whitaker RS, Simel LR, Berchuck A, Murphy SK. Quantitative detection of RASSF1A DNA promoter methylation in tumors and serum of patients with serous epithelial ovarian cancer. Gynecologic Oncology. 2011;**123**:581-587

[285] Schoofs T, Berdel WE, Muller-Tidow C. Origins of aberrant DNA methylation in acute myeloid leukemia. Leukemia. 2014;**28**:1-14

[286] Andres G, Ashour N, Sanchez-Chapado M, Ropero S, Angulo JC. The study of DNA methylation in urological cancer: Present and future. Actasurologicasespanolas. 2013;**37**:368-375

[287] Abdel-Hafiz HA, Horwitz KB. Role of epigenetic modifications in luminal breast cancer. Epigenomics. 2015;**7**:847-862

[288] Ammerpohl O, Haake A, Pellissery S, Giefing M, Richter J, Balint B, et al. Array-based DNA methylation analysis in classical Hodgkin lymphoma reveals new insights into the mechanisms underlying silencing of B cell-specific genes. Leukemia. 2012;**26**:185-188

[289] Udali S, Guarini P, Moruzzi S, Choi SW, Friso S. Cardiovascular epigenetics: From DNA methylation

to microRNAs. Molecular Aspects of Medicine. 2013;**34**:883-901

[290] Wockner LF, Noble EP, Lawford BR, Young RM, Morris CP, Whitehall VL, et al. Genome-wide DNA methylation analysis of human brain tissue from schizophrenia patients. Translational Psychiatry. 2014;**4**(339)

Chapter 3

Aflatoxins: Toxicity, Occurrences and Chronic Exposure

Bismark Dabuo, Emmanuella Wesome Avogo, Gabriel Owusu Koomson, Maxwell Akantibila and Daniel Ayendo Gbati

Abstract

Aflatoxins, a carcinogenic group of mycotoxins, are naturally occurring toxic fungi that cause illness in both animals and humans. Predominantly found in hot and humid areas, aflatoxins are generated by Aspergillus fungi and are found in a large percentage of the world's food supply. Aflatoxin B1 (AFB1), being the most potent of the over 18 aflatoxins discovered, is most noted for its role in the development of hepatocellular carcinoma (HCC) in humans and animals, unfortunately, many features of the illnesses it causes and the mechanisms that produce them, remain unexplained. This review examined AFB1 metabolism; its epoxidation and DNA adduction, its correlations to cancer initiation and the mechanisms that underpin it, the synergistic interactions with stunted growth associated with AFB1 intake and kwashiorkor, involvement of oxidative stress and reactive oxygen species. Its harmful effects, including growth retardation, starvation, and immunotoxicity, were also discussed, delving into new findings of AFB1 contamination in worldwide food sources. This review indicated that AFB1 is commonly found in high concentrations in food supplies, notably in maize. To lessen the global burden of AFB1 toxicity, data gathered through this review emphasized the necessity to apply novel and existing techniques to prevent these toxins on other diseases.

Keywords: aflatoxin, toxicology, teratogenicity, malnutrition, kwashiorkor, oxidative stress

1. Introduction

Mycotoxins are unrelated structural secondary metabolites produced by various molds, most of which belong to one of three genera; Aspergillus, Penicillium, or Fusarium [1]. There are two kinds of mycotoxin-producing fungi; field fungi, such as Fusarium species, produce mycotoxins on crops that are still growing, and storage fungi, such as Aspergillus and Penicillium species which produce mycotoxins after the crops have been harvested [2].

Aflatoxins, and being widespread in many human foods, are the biggest threat to food safety. Aflatoxins, since their discovery, have been found to be highly toxic to humans; being linked to liver cancer in humans for instance. Being common in agricultural products, such as maize, groundnut, millets, and their derivatives serving as the primary carriers, aflatoxins are prevalent in tropical and subtropical countries, posing high risks as food and feed pollutants, resulting in an excessive frequency of several deadly chronic diseases and aflatoxicosis epidemics [3].

2. Occurrence in food

The FAO's forecast for world cereal production in 2021 has been reduced by 2.1 million tonnes since November, to 2 791 million tonnes, still 0.7 percent (19.2 million tonnes) higher than the previous year's output and a new high. However, the forecast for world coarse grains production remains 1.4 percent higher on an annual basis. In the case of wheat, recent reports from Brazil and the United Kingdom of Great Britain and Northern Ireland indicating smaller harvests than expected have resulted in a slightly lower global production forecast, now pegged at 769.6 million tonnes, reinforcing an expected 1 percent year-over-year decline. In the case of rice, government estimates in Pakistan show that a record crop was harvested this season, defying FAO predictions of a minor decline in output due to water restrictions in several areas. This change, when combined with a yield-based increase for the United States of America, compensates for somewhat lower output projections in Thailand [4]. These figures demonstrate the significance of cereals and other grains in the world food supply. AFB1, on the other hand, is known to infect cereals and grains products, as well as other commonly consumed foods like groundnuts, dried fruits, and spices. The studies that found AFB1 contamination in these commodities are listed below.

2.1 Maize

Maize has the highest observed concentrations of AFB1. In Croatia, Pakistan, and the Democratic Republic of Congo, maximum AFB1 levels >1000 g/kg were discovered (2072, 1405.3, and 1401.45 μg/kg, respectively). For the investigation in the Democratic Republic of Congo, samples were evaluated after harvest, during transportation, and lastly at the market. The incidence of AFB1 infection increased considerably between freshly harvested maize (32%), and market samples (100%) [5]. Both examinations that used Pakistani samples discovered high levels of contamination. Maximum values of 1405.3 μg/kg were discovered in Lahore, Pakistan, while maximum levels of 409.3 μg/kg were discovered in Punjab, Pakistan [6]. The maize samples were collected during an unusually hot and dry season, according to the Croatian study, which could explain why the levels were so high (2072 μg /kg) [7]. In investigations into maize contamination, 46.1% of samples tested positive for AFB1, with an average maximum concentration of 553.9 μg/kg [8].

2.2 Rice

AFB1 contamination in rice has recently been identified in various Asian nations. Aflatoxin-producing fungus and aflatoxins were discovered in 187 rice samples in a Brazilian analysis. In these samples, 383 Aspergillus fungus strains were found, with 17% of those strains capable of producing type B aflatoxins. AFB1 contamination was discovered in 14% of rice samples, with AFB1 levels ranging from 0 to 63.32 μg/kg [9]. 230 rice samples were collected from various locations in Brazil during an outbreak in 2007–2009, according to another study. Many samples were contaminated with mycotoxins like ochratoxin A, deoxynivalenol, and zearalenone, and up to 180.74 g/kg of AFB1 was found [10]. AFB1 was detected in 56 of the 199 rice samples examined in Canada, with concentrations ranging from 7.1 to 7.1 μg/kg. AFB1 levels in Chinese rice ranged from 0.1 to 136.8 g/kg, with fumonisin B1 infection found in several of the samples. Ecuadorian rice samples had amounts as high as 47.4 grams per kilogram, while Iran and India reported levels as high as 6.3 and 308 grams per kilogram, respectively [11]. Three distinct investigations on rice contamination with AFB1 were conducted in Pakistan. AFB1 contamination was discovered in 35 percent, 52 percent, and 95.4 percent of the samples, with maximum AFB1 levels of 21.3, 32.9, and 24.54 μg/kg, respectively, in these three studies. Rice samples from Sweden and Malaysia were also found to be contaminated with AFB1 [11].

2.3 Wheat/Sorghum/Cereals

In a few recent studies, AFB1 has been discovered in wheat, sorghum, and cereals. Even though it was only evaluated in a few trials, sorghum had the highest average frequency of AFB1 contamination (67.3%) and the second-highest average maximum concentration (83.6 μg/kg) of all food products [12]. Wheat had the lowest average maximum concentration of 6.0 μg/kg, although having the highest AFB1 contamination rate (44.8%) [13].

2.4 Groundnuts

The contamination of groundnuts with AFB1 has been studied. Peanuts are the most commonly contaminated groundnuts; however, pistachios and hazelnuts have also been discovered to be contaminated. AFB1 was found in ten of twenty-one peanut butter samples in a Japanese study, albeit the amounts were not higher than 2.59 μg/kg. Aflatoxin contamination was not found in unprocessed peanut samples, which were also analyzed in the study [11]. The occurrence of AFB1 was investigated in three different areas of China in one study. AFB1 contamination was discovered in 100 percent of the peanut samples tested in this study, however at modest levels (up to 0.7 g/kg). Malaysia has also identified peanut contamination, with levels as high as 15.33 μg/kg. Groundnut contamination was investigated in Burkina Faso and Mozambique in a study. Burkina Faso had moderate AFB1 levels of up to 15.5 μg/kg, whilst Mozambique had high AFB1 levels of up to 123 μg/kg [11]. Turkey's groundnuts were the topic of two separate studies in 2014 and 2016. Contamination was discovered in 16.9% of the 302 samples tested in the previous study, with AFB1 levels ranging from 0.16 to 368 μg/kg. In the latter study, only 6.5 percent of the 170 samples tested positive for AFB1 contamination, with values ranging from 0.09 to 10.6 μg/kg [14]. Thailand samples revealed a low percentage of groundnut contamination (9%), whereas Zimbabwe samples had high AFB1 levels of up to 175.9 g/kg, although having a low degree of contamination (12.5%) [15].

2.5 Fruits/spices

Although fruits and spices have been studied, they are not a source of AFB1 exposure. Spices (cumin, black pepper, and chili pods/powder) had the second-highest average frequency of contamination (64.4%), as well as the highest average maximum AFB1 concentration (25.4 μg/kg) [11]. Dried fruits (such as figs, raisins, currants, sultanas, plums, dates, and apricots) had the second-lowest frequency (36.0%) and average maximum value of 16.3 μg/kg [16].

2.6 Reports of AFB1 occurrence in food commodities

Table for rice

Country	Total number of samples	Total number of positive AFB1	Mininum AFB1 levels (μg/kg)	Maximum AFB1 levels (μg/kg)	Positive percentage for AFB1	References
Brazil	187	21	Null	63.32	11.2	[10]
Pakistan	208	73	0.04	21.4	35.1	[17]
Pakistan	1027	189	1.1	32.9	18.4	[18]
Ecuador	43	3	4.9	47.4	7.0	[19]

Table for maize

Country	Total number of samples	Total number of positive AFB1	Minimum AFB1 levels	Maximum AFB1 levels	Positive percentage for AFB1	References
Democratic Republic of Congo	50 (harvest)	16	1.5	51.23	32.0	[5]
South Africa	114	15	1	133	13.2	[20]
Tanzania	Null	Null	0.53	364	29.0	[21]
Pakistan	75	73	0.5	409.3	97.3	[6]
Croatia	633	241	1.1	2072	38.1	[7]
Pakistan	100	52	2	1405.3	52.0	[18]
Mozambique	13	6	16.3	363	46.2	[22]
Burkina faso	26	13	3.4	636	50	[22]

Table for wheat

Country	Total number of samples	Total number of positive AFB1	Minimum AFB1 levels	Maximum AFB1 levels	Positive percentage for AFB1	References
China	178	11	0.03	0.12	6.2	[12]

Table for cereal

Country	Total number of samples	Total number of positive AFB1	Minimum AFB1 levels	Maximum AFB1 levels	Positive percentage for AFB1	References
Pakistan	237	98	0.04	6.9	41.1	[17]
Spain, Italy, Morocco, Tunisia	173	14	6.4	66.7	8.1	[11]

Table for Sorghum

Country	Total number of samples	Total number of positive AFB1	Minimum AFB1 levels	Maximum AFB1 levels	Positive percentage for AFB1	References
India	1606	1173	0.01	263.98	73.0	[23]
Sudan	60	17	0.06	12.29	28.3	[11]
Ethiopia	90	85	null	33.1	94.4	[13]

Table for nuts

Country	Total number of samples	Total number of positive AFB1	Minimum AFB1 levels	Maximum AFB1 levels	Positive percentage for AFB1	References
Zimbabwe	208	26	0.7	175.9	12.5	[15]
Mozambique	23	3	3.4	123	13.0	[22]
Turkey	170	11	0.09	10.6	6.5	[14]
Pakistan	180	83	0.04	14.5	46.1	[24]
Turkey	302	51	0.16	368	16.9	[25]
Thailand	25	9	0.04	4.74	36.0	[26]
Burkina Faso	9	2	5.6	15.5	22.2	

Table for spice

Country	Total number of samples	Total number of positive AFB1	Minimum AFB1 levels	Maximum AFB1 levels	Positive percentage for AFB1	References
Thailand	60	40	0.1	53.62	66.7	[26]
Italy	130	11	0.08	>15	8.5	[27]
Malaysia	58	49	0.01	28.43	84.5	[28]

Table for dried fruits

Country	Total number of samples	Total number of positive AFB1	Minimum AFB1 levels	Maximum AFB1 levels	Positive percentage for AFB1	References
Iran	88	50	0.3	8.4	56.8	[16]
Turkey	130	16	0.1	12.5	12.3	[14]
Pakistan	77	33	0.04	9.8	42.9	[24]
Greece	26	6	null	<2	23.1	[29]

3. Toxicology

Aflatoxins are a set of compounds that are very similar with tiny molecular differences. Aflatoxin B1 is the most prevalent and powerful of these poisons (AFB1). In mammals, the toxin is processed by various distinct pathways [30] . The fraction of the dose routed into the several possible pathways defines aflatoxin sensitivity across human and animal species, with harmful "biological" exposure the result of epoxide activation and epoxide interaction with proteins and DNA. There's also evidence that dosage affects the fractions that follow different possible pathways, maybe due to the saturation of the most chemically competitive processes [31]. The youth are more susceptible to Aflatoxin, and there are considerable differences across species, individuals within the same species (based on their ability to detoxify aflatoxin via biochemical mechanisms), and the sexes (according to the concentrations of testosterone). The variation in aflatoxin toxicity depends on the difference in nutritional parameters because aflatoxin exposure slows recovery from protein deficiency [32]. Aflatoxism is the term for the toxicity induced by aflatoxins. Two forms of aflatoxicosis have been identified: acute severe intoxication, which causes immediate liver damage and eventually illness or death, and chronic sub-symptomatic exposure. The dose and duration of aflatoxin exposure have a major impact on toxicity and can result in a variety of outcomes, according to a review of the literature across all species: Large doses cause acute sickness and death, primarily owing to liver cirrhosis; chronic sub-lethal doses create nutritional and immunologic issues; and all doses raise cancer risk [3] (**Figure 1**).

3.1 Mechanisms of toxicity

The majority of aflatoxins' toxicological implications and mechanisms remain unknown. An extensive study of the causes of aflatoxins' toxicity was done to provide

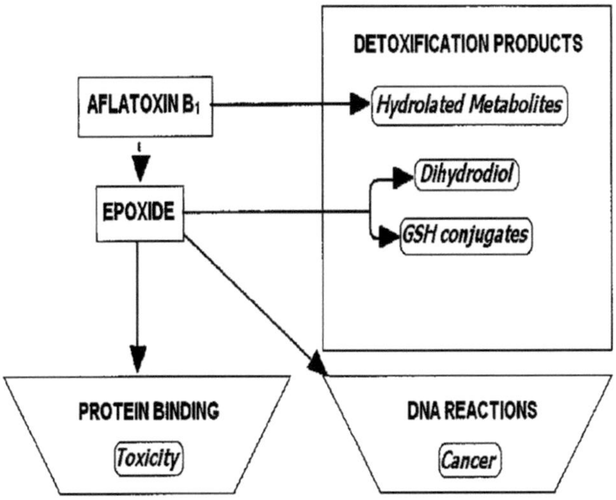

Figure 1.
Aflatoxins have a metabolic route that involves protein binding (toxicity) or DNA reactions (cancers). Hydroxylated metabolites, such as aflatoxin M1, GSH, glutathione, and the epoxide, are some of the hazardous secondary products of this system.

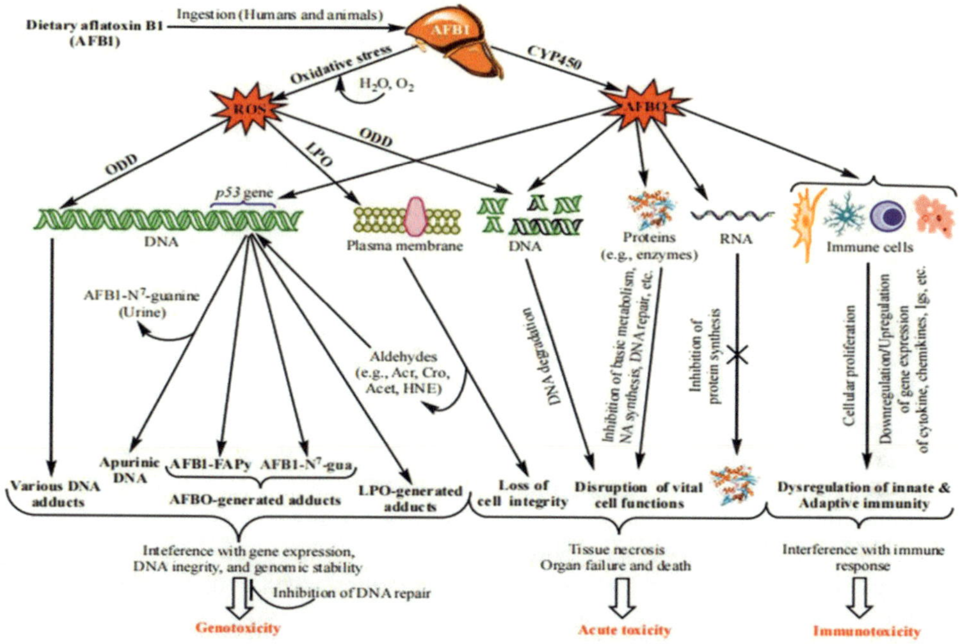

Figure 2.
Main aflatoxin B1 toxicity mechanisms are mediated by oxidative stress and AFB1-exo-8,9 epoxide. NB: ROS also affects proteins, RNA molecules, and immunity as does AFBO. Abbreviations: AFBO: Aflatoxin B1-exo-8,9-epoxide; NA: Nucleic acids; ROS: Reactive oxygen species; LPO: Lipid peroxidation; ODD: Oxidative DNA damage; Acr: Acrolein; Cro: Crotonaldehyde; Acet: Acetaldehyde; HNE: 4-Hydroxy-2-Nonenal; uFA: Unsaturated fatty acids; IL1β: Interleukin 1β, IL6: Interleukin 6; TNFα: Tumor necrotizing factor α; P-dG: Cyclic Propano-Deoxyguanosine; Igs: Immunoglobulins [3].

a scientific foundation for the development of preventive and control strategies. Authorities in charge of food safety might use a deep grasp of the subject as a scientific tool to attain regulatory objectives. The majority of study on AFB1 has focused on its mutagenesis capabilities, which have been related to the AFB1-exo-8,9 epoxide since its discovery as an intermediate metabolite (AFBO) [3]. AFBO mixes with biological macromolecules as nucleic acids, proteins, and phospholipids to affect genetic, metabolic, signaling, and cell structure [33]. However, new evidence is developing that AFB1 causing oxidative stress (OS) has an equal or higher influence on cell function and integrity [34]. **Figure 2** summarizes the AFB1 toxicity pathways that operate on genomic DNA, other functional macromolecules, and immunocompetent cells to generate genotoxicity, immunotoxicity, and acute intoxication.

3.2 Aflatoxins lead to other chronic infections

Chronic ailments result from a lifetime of low-dose aflatoxins exposure, the most prevalent and deadly of which is cancer. While aflatoxins have long been linked to primary liver malignancies including HCC and bile duct hyperplasia, they have also been linked to cancers of the kidney, pancreas, bladder, bone, and viscera [3]. Again, aflatoxins have been linked to lung and skin malignancies in workers who breathe them or come into close contact with them. Immunosuppression, teratogenicity, mutagenicity, cytotoxicity, and estrogenic effects are induced in mammals due to long-term exposure to aflatoxins. Aflatoxins have also been thought to contribute to childhood diseases such as kwashiorkor and growth failure by interfering with micronutrient absorption, protein synthesis, and metabolic enzyme performance [3].

3.3 Acute toxicity

Although the cause of acute aflatoxicosis is unknown, when aflatoxins inter relate with large biological molecules such as proteins, phospholipids, and nucleic acids, they form various adducts that interfere with the physiological and structural functions of these biological molecules. Aflatoxin-protein adducts have been related to acute intoxication because they inhibit protein synthesis, particularly enzymes implicated in essential functions such as metabolic pathways, protein synthesis, DNA replication and repair, and immunological response. There is a growing body of evidence that cell, mitochondrial, and endoplasmic reticulum membrane disruption is due to aflatoxin-phospholipid adducts and ROS-induced LPO [33]. As reported by a scientific study on AFB1's acute toxicity in chicken birds, aflatoxin–dihydrodiol (AF–dhd) is the main metabolite responsible for acute aflatoxicosis since it is the important metabolite that leads to the formation of aflatoxin–albumin adducts [35]. AFB2a has shown a covalent association with cellular proteins and phospholipids, resulting in the linkage of long-chain fatty acids and protein adducts, which may lead to acute aflatoxicosis [33]. Long-term exposure to low levels of aflatoxins, on the other hand, can cause symptoms similar to acute aflatoxicosis; however, as previously mentioned, these symptoms can be mitigated by the removal of harmful substances by phase II enzymes and cellular absorption of free radicals, as well as DNA repair to prevent mutations. Alternatively, these effects may build over time with repeated low-dose exposure, eventually leading to liver cancer as a common side effect [3]. When the dose is excessively high, a rapid rise in a short time might cause acute aflatoxicosis. Excessive amounts of aflatoxins can overwhelm the cell's detoxification capacity, driving the toxins' metabolism toward the production of toxic metabolites, resulting in severe DNA damage, cell growth disruption, asexual cloning by the DNA, metabolic disorders, cytotoxicity, and tissue necrosis, eventually leading to organ failure in a short time. This is especially important because the harmful effects of aflatoxin accumulate over time (Colakoglu and Donmez, 2012), which could lead to more devastating situations than cancers that have been more established.

3.4 Cancers caused by prolonged aflatoxin exposure

Aflatoxin has been speculated to cause liver cancer in humans, but it can also cause lung cancer in people who work with infected crops. Mutations in the tumor-suppressing gene P53, as well as the activation of dominant oncogenes, induce hepatomas [37]. The cancer risk from aflatoxin exposure has been well documented and is based on a lifetime dose [38]. The International Cancer Research Institute has categorized aflatoxin as a Class 1 carcinogen, resulting in its regulation to very low levels in traded commodities (20 ppb in grains and 0.5 ppb in milk in the United States; 4 ppb in foods in several European nations) [37]. Hepatitis B and C virus (HBV/HCV) outbreaks, on the other hand, affect roughly 20% of the population in several poor countries, appearing to have a good synergy with these biological agents for liver cancer. Aflatoxin is 30 times more potent in people with hepatitis B surface antigen than in people without the virus, and when HBV infection and aflatoxin exposure are coupled, the relative risk of cancer in HBV patients climbs from 5 to 60 [18]. In some areas where aflatoxin contamination and HBV coexist, hepatomas are the most common malignancy (64 percent of malignancies; 25) and may be the primary cause of mortality.

Aflatoxin B1 is expected to cause between 25,200 and 155,000 cases of liver cancer per year, with 40% of cases occurring in Sub-Saharan Africa, where aflatoxin-induced liver cancer accounts for one-third of all liver cancer occurrences [39]. Aflatoxin B1 is expected to cause between 25,200 and 155,000 cases of liver cancer per year, with 40% of cases occurring in Sub-Saharan Africa, where aflatoxin-induced liver cancer accounts for one-third of all liver cancer occurrences [40].

3.5 Teratogenicity

Aflatoxin exposure in pregnant women or birds can affect unfertilized eggs or embryos in utero, resulting in a variety of poor health effects and abnormal gestation/incubation outcomes [41]. Aflatoxin or its metabolites are transmitted to the infant during pregnancy and processed using the same mechanisms as adults [42]. In pregnant women, it has been demonstrated by scientific kinds of literature that, aflatoxins can be transferred from mothers to offspring through blood circulations. In fetal cord blood and maternal blood samples, aflatoxin metabolites, aflatoxin-DNA, and aflatoxin–albumin adducts, as well as biomarkers derived from them, were found [42]. As a result, fetal growth restriction, fetal loss, or premature birth may occur in significantly exposed mothers' pregnancies. An adverse association between birth weight and the levels of suitable biomarkers in the cord blood has been extensively documented in people and animals when growth restriction is present [43]. However, little research has shown excess aflatoxin accumulations by pregnant women to stillbirth, and research on the link between excess aflatoxin consumption by pregnant women and premature birth and fetal loss is confusing or contradictory [44]. Furthermore, an enriched aflatoxin diet harms pregnant women's state of complete physical, mental and social well-being and exposes their fetuses to congenital defects as a result of indirect impacts. Increased systemic inflammation, for example, is caused by overexpression of maternal pro-inflammatory cytokines and/or downregulation of anti-inflammatory cytokines, which affects and causes placental insufficiency, resulting in poor fetal growth, miscarriage, stillbirth, or premature birth [41]. Anemia and high aflatoxin intake were found to be linked in a cross-sectional study of Ghanaian women, as evaluated by the AFB-albumin adduct in the mothers' serum [45]. However, there is no evidence of a relationship between aflatoxins exposure and inflammation-induced anemia in pregnant women [3].

3.6 Genotoxicity caused by oxidative stress

Although the creation of aflatoxin-N7-gua DNA adducts has been attributed to the majority of aflatoxins' mutagenicity, it is becoming clear that oxidative stress (OS) created by AFB1 metabolism is also a role [46]. The OS can cause oxidative DNA damage (ODD) either directly on DNA or indirectly through membrane phospholipid lipid peroxidation by-products (LPO). OS is caused by the release of large amounts of reactive oxygen species (ROS) from the breakdown of AFB1 by CYP450 enzymes in the liver, which can damage DNA's nitrogen bases and deoxyribose moieties, resulting in in in over 100 distinct DNA adducts [3]. The most well-known and examined of these adducts is 7,8-dihydro-8-oxo-20-deoxyguanosine (8-hydroxydeoxyguanosine, 8-oxo-dG, 8-OH-dG), which is commonly employed as a biomarker for oxidative DNA damage [3]. Intraperitoneal injection of AFB1 into rats elevated 8-oxo-dG levels in the liver in a dose- and time-dependent manner, which was avoided by pre-treatment of animals with the antioxidants selenium and deferoxamine, establishing the relationship between the adduct and Aflatoxin-induced oxidative stress [3]. latest scientific work found no notable increase in seven ROS-modified bases in the liver tissues of rats treated with 7.5 mg/kg AFB1, including 8-oxo-dG, when compared to control rats (untreated); however, levels of 8,50 -cyclo-20 -deoxyadenosine, another DNA adduct from the oxidative attack of the adenine base, increased significantly [47]. By organisms, organs, tissue, sub-cellular component, and cell cycle, the quantity of oxidative DNA damage, the kind of adduct produced, and the effectiveness and speed of DNA repair have all been found to differ [3]. AFG1 increased the expression of tumor necrosis factor (TNF)- and CYP2A13 in mouse alveolar type II (AT-II) cells of lung tissues, as well as in vitro in human AT-II-like cells (A549), which mediate inflammation by increasing the number of -H2AX- and 8-OHdG-positive cells in inflamed tissues, according to a recent scientific study [48]. The inflammatory response generated by TNF increases the expression of CYP2A13, which keeps AFG1 active and causes ODD, as seen by increased expression of the DNA damage marker -H2AX. GT transversion mutations are caused by 8-oxo-dG lesions, which are similar to AFBO-derived DNA adducts but do not pick out the p53 gene and necessitate the use of additional processes and DNA polymerases [35].

3.7 Aflatoxins and the immune system's relationship

Reduced vaccination efficacy, evidence of aflatoxins affecting both innate and acquired/adaptive immunity was found to have an increased incidence and severity of infectious infections, as well as prolonged healing times [3]. According to a study, AFB1 immunotoxicity is mediated by AFBO, as well as interchanging with immunocompetent cells throughout the body, altering their fast growth and/or the manufacture of immune reaction mediators, disrupting innate and adaptive immunity. Although these mechanisms were established using animal studies, AFB1's immunotoxicity has also been confirmed in vitro on human cell lines and in case–control studies in heavily exposed areas such as Ghana [3, 49]. In rats, a ten-fold higher dose of 1 mg AFB1/kg bw increased the number of CD8+ (cytotoxic T cells) while not affecting other immunological markers [3]. Other scientific studies, on the other hand, have demonstrated that the immune response can be altered even at low levels of aflatoxins and shorter exposure times. For example, rats were fed a portion of food that contain about 5 to 75 g AFB1/kg bw for five weeks [50], Other research, on the other hand, has demonstrated that the immune response can be altered even at low levels of aflatoxins and shorter exposure intervals. For five weeks, rats were fed a diet with 5 to 75 g AFB1/kg bw [51]. Although the preponderance of evidence suggests that aflatoxins mostly impair immune function, in vitro and in vivo investigations have revealed that they can also dysregulate immune responses through immunostimulatory effects [52].

3.8 The link between aflatoxins and innate immunity

In vivo and in vitro, structurally barriers example: skin and intestinal epithelial cells are damaged, causing the weakened structure–function against microbial and toxin intrusions. The production of intra-epidermal vesicles and squamous cell carcinoma have been connected to contact with the skin of a variety of animals [53]. Pigs fed an aflatoxins-contaminated diet for 28 days exhibited crusting and skin ulceration on their snouts, lips, and buccal commissures (AFB1, AFB2, AFG1, and AFG2) [3]. Aflatoxins have been shown to impair the intestine's mechanical barrier by interrupting cell cycle development or damaging intestinal epithelial cells and the tight junctions that hold them together in scientific review studies. Broilers fed 0.6 mg AFB1/kg food for exactly 3 weeks had their cell growth interrupted at the G2/M phase, leading to a decrease in jejunum height and a decrease in the villus height/crypt ratio, jeopardizing their function as a selective barrier [54]. The mechanical, chemical, and immunological barriers that protect the gut mucosa from external assaults at the molecular level are affected by aflatoxins. The CacO-2 human cell line was treated in vitro with 1–100 M AFB1 for 48 hours, which decreased trans-epithelial electrical resistance (TEER). As a result, paracellular permeability increased and survival decreased [55]. After 48 hours of exposure to varying doses of AFM1, CacO-2 cells' selective permeability was likewise impaired (0.2 to 20 M) [56]. Cell viability, function, or gene expression of cytokines and chemokines in immune cells like monocytes, macrophages, dendritic cells (DC), and natural killer (NK) cells, all of which play important roles in innate immunity has been shown by a certain secondary metabolite (Flavonoids). TLR-2, TLR-4, and TLR-7 transcription are suppressed in broilers exposed to AFB1, showing a suppressive effect on innate immunity. These receptor proteins have a role in sentinel cells like macrophages and dendritic cells recognizing external invaders, which is a crucial step in initiating an immune response [57]. Human monocytes were pre-treated for 24 hours with as little as 0.1 pg. AFB1/mL before being cultured with *Candida albicans* for 30 minutes at 37°C [3]. In addition, the aflatoxins AFB1, AFB2, and/or AFM1 have been shown in other studies to reduce macrophage viability, proliferation, cytotoxicity, and phagocytic activity, as well as the expression of cytokines like TNF-, IL-1, and IL-6, and the inducible nitric oxide synthase (iNOS), which mediate intracellular pathogen killing during phagocytosis [3]. When dairy cow neutrophils were given low doses of AFB1 for 18 hours (0.01, 0.05, and 0.5 ng/mL), their phagocytic and cytotoxic capacities against *Staphylococcus aureus* and *Escherichia coli* were drastically diminished. This was attributed to the reduction of reactive oxygen species (ROS) in neutrophil cytoplasm, which is important for pathogen killing during phagocytosis [58]. In numerous mammals, aflatoxins blocked the complement system, which is a critical component of innate defense that causes the phagocytosis of dangerous microorganisms [3]. Complement activity was observed to be decreased in cattle and poultry fed at varying threshold levels [59]. After ducklings were fed AFB1 at doses of 0.5 or 0.8 mg/kg feed for 40 days, the APCA was activated for the first 15 days, then suppressed for the remaining days of the study. In contrast, the effect of aflatoxins on the complement system appears to be very reliant on the host, as rabbits fed a 24 mg/kg diet for 28 days showed no significant change in serum hemolytic activity (CH50) [3].

3.9 The link between aflatoxins and adaptive immunity

The decrease of adaptive/acquired immunity that occurs as a result of aflatoxins exposure is well documented, implying that exposed hosts are more susceptible to infectious pathogens and that vaccine protection is reduced or nonexistent [60]. In contrast to a control group fed an aflatoxin-free diet, vaccination failed to protect pigs against *Erysipelothrix rhusiopathiae* when fed AFB1-contaminated feed [3]. Humans and animals have shown reduced lymphocyte fast growth, activation, and/or function. In adaptive immunity, lymphocytes are the most significant immune cells. Apoptosis was seen in human peripheral blood cells treated at diverse times with different dosages of AFG1 (3.12–2000 g/L) [61]. In vitro treatment of human lymphocytes with AFB1 at concentrations ranging from 5 to 165 uM increased the frequency of apoptotic and necrotic lymphocytes in a dose-dependent manner, with a considerable increase in cell necrosis beginning at 50 uM (15.6 mg/L) after 24 hours [62]. T-cell proliferation was decreased in a dose-dependent manner starting at 15 M in vitro culture of the human lymphoblastoid Jurkat T-cell line with AFB1 or AFM1 at 3-50 M concentrations range for 72 hours, but no apoptosis or necrosis was seen [63]. When compared to negative control cells cultivated in the absence of aflatoxins, AFB1 and AFM1 dramatically enhanced the expression of IL-8, a cytokine implicated in innate immunity, while adaptive immunity was unaffected, as seen by unchanged levels of interferon (INF)- and IL-2 cytokine [3]. AFB1 and AFM1 significantly increased the expression of IL-8, a cytokine implicated in innate immunity, when compared to negative control cells cultivated in the absence of aflatoxins, while adaptive immunity was unaffected, as seen by unchanged levels of interferon (INF)- and IL-2 cytokine [64]. The suppression of adaptive CMI has been researched in lab animals such as chickens and rats, with results showing a decrease in the amount of distinct T-cell lymphocyte subsets as well as the cytokines they release, both of which are important components of this form of the immune response. Reduced delayed-type hypersensitivity (DTH) in a variety of species, including chicken and rats, at doses ranging from 0.3 to 1.0 mg/kg feed, supported adaptive CMI suppression by aflatoxins, meaning a reduction in the frequency of adaptive CMI cases [65]. Rats given AFB1 dosages ranging from 5 to 75 g/kg bw for five weeks had decreased proliferation and cytokine production in splenic helper T cells (CD4+) engaging in acquired cellular immunity. In laboratory animals, adaptive CMI has been studied [50]. AFM1 decreased DTH and related T lymphocyte subsets (CD3+, CD4+, CD8+, CD19+, and CD49 b), as well as the interleukins they release, such as INF-, IL-10, and IL-4, in mice administered 25 or 50 g/kg bw intraperitoneally [49]. A decrease in CD3+ and CD19+ lymphocyte subsets bearing the D69 activation marker (i.e., CD3 + CD69+ and CD19 + CD69+), as well as CD8+ T-cells, which play a key role in vaccination and immune response against pathogens, was highly correlated with high levels of AFB1, as measured by the concentrations of AFB1-albumin adduct in the serum [66].

3.10 Aflatoxins, malnutrition, and neurodegenerative diseases are linked

Aflatoxins have been linked to a variety of diseases, each with its own set of processes and risk factors. Malnutrition problems include malnutrition (faltering and stunting), physical and mental maturation issues, reproductive and sexuality troubles, and nervous system abnormalities, among others (neurodegenerative diseases and neuroblastoma) [67, 68]. Chronic aflatoxins exposure has been related to neurological illnesses, according to a growing body of scientific evidence. In neuronal brain cells, oxidative stress caused by aflatoxins, as well as AFBO and ROS produced by CYP450 enzymes, react with functional macromolecules, restricting lipid and protein synthesis and causing degeneration [69]. Aflatoxins have also been shown to disrupt the structure and function of mitochondria in brain cells, causing oxidative phosphorylation to be inhibited and cell [70]. As with vitamins A, C, and E, aflatoxin interferes with vitamin and mineral absorption, worsening low nutritional status, and selenium deficiency inhibits children's growth [71]. As a result, children exposed during pregnancy may develop growth abnormalities that remain throughout adulthood, including stunted and delayed physical and mental maturation [72].

3.11 Aflatoxin and kwashiorkor investigations in the past

A possible link between aflatoxin exposure and childhood kwashiorkor, a disorder characterized by the protein-energy shortage, was debated decades ago. Kwashiorkor and marasmus (another malnutrition-related childhood disease prevalent in impoverished countries) are both severe malnutrition diseases. Although protein deficiency is a fundamental cause of both kwashiorkor and marasmus, one key difference between the two conditions is that kwashiorkor can occur even when the children's calorie intake is adequate, whereas marasmus can only be caused by low caloric intake [73]. Fatty liver and edema, both frequent kwashiorkor signs, are less likely in children with marasmus. Kwashiorkor's symptoms include anorexia and light-colored hair and skin [74]. Marasmic kwashiorkor is defined as edema from kwashiorkor combined with wasting from marasmus [75]. According to a scientific study, children with kwashiorkor had higher amounts of aflatoxins or their metabolites in their blood or urine than children with other protein malnutrition-related illnesses such as marasmus. Furthermore, aflatoxins were identified in autopsies of children who died from kwashiorkor in their lungs and livers, but not in their kidneys, but not at statistically significant levels, compared to those who died from other diseases or other forms of malnutrition [76]. Kwashiorkor patients were paired with children who did not show any indications or symptoms of protein-energy deficit. All of the children's serum and/or urine contained aflatoxins. Although the controls had a higher proportion of urine aflatoxins than the kwashiorkor group, the kwashiorkor group had a much higher serum/urine ratio. Rather than aflatoxin playing a direct role in the production of kwashiorkor, these data could imply that kwashiorkor has decreased liver function, which could lead to abnormalities in aflatoxin metabolism. Indeed, it has been proposed that children with kwashiorkor are more susceptible to the hazards of Aflatoxin in the diet [74].

4. Conclusions

Aflatoxins being very common and highly toxic, pose a great threat to food safety, more research would aid in a better understanding of their toxicity incidence, patterns, and resultant correlations with foods and other illnesses to appropriately address their negative effects on public health and the economy. With the growing prevalence of aflatoxin in developing countries where agroclimatic zones encourage aflatoxin growth in cash crops such as peanut, maize, sorghum, and sunflower; contamination of farm produce in endemic regions continues to be a major impediment to international trade and food security, as it not only affects local populations but also has the potential to spread to other parts of the world by either exporting highly contaminated goods or restricting their marketability, both of which contribute to rising prices and limiting access. Interventions can be made to target the inhibitions of these fungi on the field and in their storage produce if the mechanism of actions is well understood. The data presented through this research aims to delve more into the growing body of evidence associating teratogenicity, immunotoxicity, malnutrition ('kwashiorkor'), neurological disease, and aflatoxin exposure with respect to cancers. More research is needed to determine the mechanism that connects aflatoxins to the many diseases they cause. The link between Aflatoxin exposure and the immune system reveals that this fugal's effect is lethal and should be handled with prudence. Furthermore, studies show that aflatoxins impair immune function in humans who are exposed to these natural fungal toxins.

Author details

Bismark Dabuo[1*], Emmanuella Wesome Avogo[2], Gabriel Owusu Koomson[3], Maxwell Akantibila[4] and Daniel Ayendo Gbati[1]

1 Department of Applied Chemistry and Biochemistry, University for Development Studies, Ghana

2 Ghana Standard Authority, Metallic Contaminant Laboratory, Ghana

3 Department of Theoretical and Applied Biology, Kwame Nkrumah University of Science and Technology, Ghana

4 Department of Biochemistry and Forensic Science, C.K. Tedam University of Technology and Applied Sciences, Ghana

*Address all correspondence to: bismarkdabuo98@gmail.com

References

[1] Greeff-Laubscher MR, Beukes I, Marais GJ, Jacobs K. Mycotoxin production by three different toxigenic fungi genera on formulated abalone feed and the effect of an aquatic environment on fumonisins. Mycology. 2020;**11**(2):105-117. DOI: 10.1080/21501203.2019.1604575

[2] Antonissen G, Martel A, Pasmans F, Ducatelle R, Verbrugghe E, Vandenbroucke V, et al. The impact of Fusarium Mycotoxins on human and animal host susceptibility to infectious diseases. Toxins. 2014;**6**(2):430-452

[3] Benkerroum N. Chronic and acute toxicities of aflatoxins: Mechanisms of action. International Journal of Environmental Research and Public Health. 2020;**17**(2):1-28

[4] Food and Agriculture Organization of the United Nation. Crop prospects and food situation. In: Crop Prospects and Food Situation. December 2021. DOI: 10.4060/cb7877en

[5] Udomkun P, Mutegi C, Wossen T, Atehnkeng J, Nabahungu NL, Njukwe E, et al. Occurrence of aflatoxin in agricultural produce from local markets in Burundi and Eastern Democratic Republic of Congo. Food Science and Nutrition. 2018;**6**(8):2227-2238. DOI: 10.1002/fsn3.787

[6] Iram W, Anjum T, Abbas M, Khan AM. Aflatoxins and ochratoxin A in maize of Punjab, Pakistan. Food Additives and Contaminants: Part B Surveillance. 2014;7(1):57-62. DOI: 10.1080/19393210.2013.843205

[7] Pleadin J, Vulić A, Perši N, Škrivanko M, Capek B, Cvetnić Ž. Aflatoxin B1 occurrence in maize sampled from Croatian farms and feed factories during 2013. Food Control. 2014;**40**(1):286-291. DOI: 10.1016/j.foodcont.2013.12.022

[8] Hofgaard IS, Brurberg MB, Sulyok M, Tronsmo AM. Multimycotoxin and fungal analysis of maize grains from south and southwestern Ethiopia. Food Additives and Contaminants: Part B Surveillance. 2017;**11**(1):64-74. DOI: 10.1080/19393210.2017.1408698

[9] Katsurayama, AM, Martins, LM, Iamanaka, BT, Fungaro, MHP, Silva, JJ, Frisvad, JC, et al. Occurrence of Aspergillus section Flavi and aflatoxins in Brazilian rice: From field to market. International Journal of Food Microbiology. 2018;**266**:213-221. DOI: 10.1016/j.ijfoodmicro.2017.12.008

[10] Almeida MI, Almeida NG, Carvalho KL, Gonçalves GAA, Silva CN, Santos EA, et al. Co-occurrence of aflatoxins B1, B2, G1 and G2, ochratoxin A, zearalenone, deoxynivalenol, and citreoviridin in rice in Brazil. Food Additives and Contaminants - Part A Chemistry, Analysis, Control, Exposure and Risk Assessment. 2012a;**29**(4):694-703

[11] Rushing BR, Selim MI. Aflatoxin B1: A review on metabolism, toxicity, occurrence in food, occupational exposure, and detoxification methods. Food and Chemical Toxicology. 2019;**124**:81-100. DOI: 10.1016/j.fct.2018.11.047

[12] Zhao Y, Wang Q, Huang J, Ma L, Chen Z, Wang F. Aflatoxin B1 and sterigmatocystin in wheat and wheat products from supermarkets in China. Food Additives and Contaminants: Part B Surveillance. 2018;**11**(1):9-14. DOI: 10.1080/19393210.2017.1388295

[13] Taye W, Ayalew A, Chala A, Dejene M. Aflatoxin B1 and total fumonisin contamination and their producing fungi in fresh and stored sorghum grain in East Hararghe, Ethiopia. Food Additives and Contaminants: Part B Surveillance. 2016;**9**(4):237-245. DOI: 10.1080/19393210.2016.1184190

[14] Kabak B. Aflatoxins in hazelnuts and dried figs: Occurrence and exposure assessment. Food Chemistry. 2016;**211**:8-16. DOI: 10.1016/j.foodchem.2016.04.141

[15] Nleya N, Adetunji MC, Mwanza M. Current status of mycotoxin contamination of food commodities in Zimbabwe. Toxins. 2018;**10**(5):1-12. DOI: 10.3390/toxins10050089

[16] Heshmati A, Zohrevand T, Khaneghah AM, Mozaffari Nejad AS, Sant'Ana AS. Co-occurrence of aflatoxins and ochratoxin A in dried fruits in Iran: Dietary exposure risk assessment. Food and Chemical Toxicology. 2017;**106**:202-208. DOI: 10.1016/j.fct.2017.05.046

[17] Iqbal SZ, Asi MR, Hanif U, Zuber M, Jinap S. The presence of aflatoxins and ochratoxin A in rice and rice products; And evaluation of dietary intake. Food Chemistry. 2016;**210**:135-140. DOI: 10.1016/j.foodchem.2016.04.104

[18] Elmore SE, Treviño-Espinosa RS, Garcia-Mazcorro JF, González-Barranco P, Sánchez-Casas RM, Phillips TD, et al. Evaluation of aflatoxin and fumonisin co-exposure in urine samples from healthy volunteers in northern Mexico. Toxicology Reports. 2021;**8**(October):1734-1741. DOI: 10.1016/j.toxrep.2021.10.001

[19] Ortiz J, Van Camp J, Mestdagh F, Donoso S, De Meulenaer B. Mycotoxin co-occurrence in rice, oat flakes and wheat noodles used as staple foods in Ecuador. Food Additives and Contaminants - Part A Chemistry, Analysis, Control, Exposure and Risk Assessment. 2013;**30**(12):2165-2176. DOI: 10.1080/19440049.2013.853228

[20] Mngqawa P, Shephard GS, Green IR, Ngobeni SH, de Rijk TC, Katerere DR. Mycotoxin contamination of home-grown maize in rural northern South Africa (Limpopo and Mpumalanga Provinces). Food Additives and Contaminants: Part B Surveillance. 2016;**9**(1):38-45. DOI: 10.1080/19393210.2015.1121928

[21] Kimanya ME, Shirima CP, Magoha H, Shewiyo DH, De Meulenaer B, Kolsteren P, et al. Co-exposures of aflatoxins with deoxynivalenol and fumonisins from maize based complementary foods in Rombo, Northern Tanzania. Food Control. 2014;**41**(1):76-81. DOI: 10.1016/j.foodcont.2013.12.034

[22] Warth B, Parich A, Atehnkeng J, Bandyopadhyay R, Schuhmacher R, Sulyok M, et al. Quantitation of mycotoxins in food and feed from burkina faso and mozambique using a modern LC-MS/MS multitoxin method. Journal of Agricultural and Food Chemistry. 2012;**60**(36):9352-9363. DOI: 10.1021/jf302003n

[23] Ratnavathi CV, Komala VV, Kumar BSV, Das IK, Patil JV. Natural occurrence of aflatoxin B1 in sorghum grown in different geographical regions of India. Journal of the Science of Food and Agriculture. 2012;**92**(12):2416-2420. DOI: 10.1002/jsfa.5646

[24] Kumar A, Pathak H, Bhadauria S, Sudan J. Aflatoxin contamination in food crops: Causes, detection, and management: A review. Food Production, Processing and Nutrition. 2021;**3**(1):2-19. DOI: 10.1186/s43014-021-00064-y

[25] Hepsag F, Golge O, Kabak B. Quantitation of aflatoxins in pistachios

and groundnuts using HPLC-FLD method. Food Control. 2014;**38**(1):75-81. DOI: 10.1016/j.foodcont.2013.10.005

[26] Tansakul N, Limsuwan S, Böhm J, Hollmann M, Razzazi-Fazeli E. Aflatoxins in selected Thai commodities. Food Additives and Contaminants: Part B Surveillance. 2013;**6**(4):254-259. DOI: 10.1080/19393210.2013.812148

[27] Mahato DK, Lee KE, Kamle M, Devi S, Dewangan KN, Kumar P, et al. Aflatoxins in food and feed: An overview on prevalence, detection and control strategies. Frontiers in Microbiology. 2019;**10**:1-10. DOI: 10.3389/fmicb.2019.02266

[28] Ali N, Hashim NH, Shuib NS. Natural occurrence of aflatoxins and ochratoxin A in processed spices marketed in Malaysia. Food Additives and Contaminants - Part A Chemistry, Analysis, Control, Exposure and Risk Assessment. 2015;**32**(4):518-532

[29] Kollia E, Kanapitsas A, Markaki P. Occurrence of aflatoxin B1 and ochratoxin A in dried vine fruits from Greek market. Food Additives and Contaminants: Part B Surveillance. 2014;**7**(1):11-16. DOI: 10.1080/19393210.2013.825647

[30] Rotimi OA, Rotimi SO, Goodrich JM, Adelani IB, Agbonihale E, Talabi, G. Time-course effects of acute aflatoxin B1 exposure on hepatic mitochondrial lipids and oxidative stress in rats. Frontiers in Pharmacology. 2019;**10**:1-10. DOI: 10.3389/fphar.2019.00467

[31] Serraino A, Bonilauri P, Kerekes K, Farkas Z, Giacometti F, Canever A, et al. Occurrence of aflatoxin M1 in raw milk marketed in Italy: Exposure assessment and risk characterization. Frontiers in Microbiology. 2019;**10**:10. DOI: 10.3389/fmicb.2019.02516

[32] Bbosa GS, Kitya D, Lubega A, Ogwal-Okeng J, WWA, DBK. Review of the biological and health effects of aflatoxins on body organs and body systems. Aflatoxins - Recent Advances and Future Prospects. 2013. p. 12-14. DOI: 10.5772/51201

[33] Rushing BR, Selim MI. Structure and oxidation of pyrrole adducts formed between Aflatoxin B2a and biological amines. Chemical Research in Toxicology. 2017;**30**(6):1275-1285. DOI: 10.1021/acs.chemrestox.7b00002

[34] Ayala A, Muñoz MF, Argüelles S. Lipid peroxidation: Production, metabolism, and signaling mechanisms of malondialdehyde and 4-hydroxy-2-nonenal. Oxidative Medicine and Cellular Longevity. 2014;**98**:9-12

[35] Diaz GJ, Murcia HW. An unusually high production of hepatic aflatoxin B1-dihydrodiol, the possible explanation for the high susceptibility of ducks to aflatoxin B1. Scientific Reports. 2019;**9**(1):18-21. DOI: 10.1038/s41598-019-44515-6

[36] Colakoglu F, Donmez HH. Effects of aflatoxin on liver and protective effectiveness of esterified glucomannan in merino rams. The Scientific World Journal. 2012;**2012**:1-5. DOI: 10.1100/2012/462925

[37] De Fromentel CC, Levrero M. P53 functional loss, stemness and hepatocellular carcinoma. Hepatoma Research. 2020;**80**:2-19

[38] Magnussen A, Parsi MA. Aflatoxins, hepatocellular carcinoma and public health. World Journal of Gastroenterology. 2013;**19**(10):1508-1512. DOI: 10.3748/wjg.v19.i10.1508

[39] Sarma UP, Bhetaria PJ, Devi P, Varma A. Aflatoxins: Implications on

health. Indian Journal of Clinical Biochemistry. 2017;**32**(2):124-133. DOI: 10.1007/s12291-017-0649-2

[40] Yang WS, Zeng XF, Liu ZN, Zhao QH, Tan YT, Gao J, et al. Diet and liver cancer risk: A narrative review of epidemiological evidence. British Journal of Nutrition. 2020;**124**(3):330-340. DOI: 10.1017/S0007114520001208

[41] Smith LE, Prendergast AJ, Turner PC, Humphrey JH, Stoltzfus RJ. Aflatoxin exposure during pregnancy, maternal anemia, and adverse birth outcomes. American Journal of Tropical Medicine and Hygiene. 2017;**96**(4):770-776. DOI: 10.4269/ajtmh.16-0730

[42] Chawanthayatham S, Thiantanawat A, Egner PA, Groopman JD, Wogan GN, Croy RG, Essigmann JM. Prenatal exposure of mice to the human liver carcinogen aflatoxin B1 reveals a critical window of susceptibility to genetic change. International Journal of Cancer. 2015;**136**(6):1254-1262. DOI: 10.1002/ijc.29102

[43] Güthle M, Dollinger MM. Epidemiology and risk factors of hepatocellular carcinoma. Der Radiologe. 2014;**54**(7):654-659. DOI: 10.1007/s00117-014-2650-6

[44] Malhotra A, Allison BJ, Castillo-Melendez M, Jenkin G, Polglase GR, Miller SL. Neonatal morbidities of fetal growth restriction: Pathophysiology and impact. Frontiers in Endocrinology. 2019;**10**(FEB):1-18. DOI: 10.3389/fendo.2019.00055

[45] Tshalibe RS. The effect of mycotoxin exposure on the growth of infants and young children in deep rural areas of the Eastern Cape Province, South Africa. 25753053. 2019. http://repository.nwu.ac.za/handle/10394/33535

[46] Ignatov AV, Bondarenko KA, Makarova AV. Non-bulky lesions in human DNA: The ways of formation, repair, and replication. Acta Naturae. 2017;**9**(3):12-26

[47] Coskun E, Jaruga P, Vartanian V, Erdem O, Egner PA, Groopman JD, et al. Aflatoxin-Guanine DNA adducts and oxidatively induced DNA damage in aflatoxin-treated mice in vivo as measured by liquid chromatography-tandem mass spectrometry with isotope dilution. Chemical Research in Toxicology. 2019;**32**(1):80-89

[48] Shao P, Guo N, Wang C, Zhao M, Yi L, Liu C, et al. Aflatoxin G1 induced TNF-α-dependent lung inflammation to enhance DNA damage in alveolar epithelial cells. Journal of Cellular Physiology. 2019;**234**(6):9194-9206. DOI: 10.1002/jcp.27596

[49] Shirani K, Zanjani BR, Mahmoudi M, Jafarian AH, Hassani FV, Giesy JP, et al. Immunotoxicity of aflatoxin M1: As a potent suppressor of innate and acquired immune systems in a subacute study. Journal of the Science of Food and Agriculture. 2018;**98**(15):5884-5892. DOI: 10.1002/jsfa.9240

[50] Qian G, Tang L, Guo X, Wang F, Massey ME, Su J, et al. Aflatoxin B1 modulates the expression of phenotypic markers and cytokines by splenic lymphocytes of male F344 rats. Journal of Applied Toxicology. 2014;**34**(3):241-249. DOI: 10.1002/jat.2866

[51] Tudek B, Zdżalik-Bielecka D, Tudek A, Kosicki K, Fabisiewicz A, Speina E. Lipid peroxidation in face of DNA damage, DNA repair and other cellular processes. Free Radical Biology and Medicine. 2017;**107**(September):77-89. DOI: 10.1016/j.freeradbiomed.2016.11.043

[52] Wang Q, Zhang Y, Zheng N, Guo L, Song X, Zhao S, et al. Biological system responses of dairy cows to aflatoxin b1 exposure revealed with metabolomic changes in multiple biofluids. Toxins. 2019;**11**(2):1-22. DOI: 10.3390/toxins11020077

[53] Gao Y, Meng L, Liu H, Wang J, Zheng N. The compromised intestinal barrier induced. Toxins. 8 september 2020. p. 1-42

[54] Yin H, Jiang M, Peng X, Cui H, Zhou Y, He M, et al. The molecular mechanism of G2/M cell cycle arrest induced by AFB1 in the jejunum. Oncotarget. 2016;**7**(24):35592-35606

[55] Romero A, Ares I, Ramos E, Castellano V, Martínez M, Martínez-Larrañaga MR, et al. Mycotoxins modify the barrier function of Caco-2 cells through differential gene expression of specific claudin isoforms: Protective effect of illite mineral clay. Toxicology. 2016;**353-354**:21-33. DOI: 10.1016/j.tox.2016.05.003

[56] Gao Y, Li S, Wang J, Luo C, Zhao S, Zheng N. Modulation of intestinal epithelial permeability in differentiated caco-2 cells exposed to aflatoxin M1 and ochratoxin a individually or collectively. Toxins. 2018;**10**(1):1-19. DOI: 10.3390/toxins10010013

[57] Wang F, Zuo Z, Chen K, Gao C, Yang Z, Zhao S, et al. Histopathological injuries, ultrastructural changes, and depressed TLR expression in the small intestine of broiler chickens with aflatoxin B1. Toxins. 2018;**10**(4):1-16. DOI: 10.3390/toxins10040131

[58] Zon G. Recent advances in aptamer applications for analytical biochemistry. Analytical Biochemistry. 2022;**644**:113894. DOI: 10.1016/j.ab.2020.113894

[59] Mehrzad J, Fazel F, Pouyamehr N, Hosseinkhani S, Dehghani H. Naturally occurring level of aflatoxin B1 injures human, canine and bovine leukocytes through ATP depletion and caspase activation. International Journal of Toxicology. 2020;**39**(1):30-38. DOI: 10.1177/1091581819892613

[60] Mohsenzadeh MS, Hedayati N, Riahi-Zanjani B, Karimi G. Immunosuppression following dietary aflatoxin B1 exposure: A review of the existing evidence. Toxin Reviews. 2016;**35**(3-4):121-127. DOI: 10.1080/15569543.2016.1209523

[61] Chen X, Horn N, Cotter PF, Applegate TJ. Growth, serum biochemistry, complement activity, and liver gene expression responses of Pekin ducklings to graded levels of cultured aflatoxin B 1. Poultry Science. 2014;**93**(8):2028-2036

[62] Al-Hammadi S, Marzouqi F, Al-Mansouri A, Shahin A, Al-Shamsi M, Mensah-Brown E, et al. The cytotoxicity of aflatoxin B1 in human lymphocytes. Sultan Qaboos University Medical Journal. 2014;**14**(1):65-71

[63] Luongo D, Russo R, Balestrieri A, Marzocco S, Bergamo P, Severino L. In vitro study of AFB1 and AFM1 effects on human lymphoblastoid Jurkat T-cell model. Journal of Immunotoxicology. 2014;**11**(4):353-358. DOI: 10.3109/1547691X.2013.848250

[64] Loftus J. Mycotoxins - an analysis of their immunomodulatory effects and methods for their detection. [thesis]. School of Biotechnology, Dublin City University; 2018. pp. 4-200

[65] Chen Xi. Impact of dietary modification on aflatoxicosis in poultry. Open Access Dissertations. 2016. p. 634.

Available from: https://docs.lib.purdue.edu/open_access_dissertations/634

[66] Chu Y, Yang H, Wu H, Liu J, Wang L, Lu S. HHS Public Access. International Journal of Cancer. 2018;**141**(1):711 720

[67] Khoury DEl, Fayjaloun S, Nassar M, Sahakian J, Aad PY. Updates on the effect of mycotoxins on male reproductive efficiency in mammals. Toxins. 2019;**11**(9):2-21. DOI: 10.3390/toxins11090515

[68] Palliyaguru DL, Wu F. Global geographical overlap of aflatoxin and hepatitis C: Controlling risk factors for liver cancer worldwide. Food Additives and Contaminants - Part A Chemistry, Analysis, Control, Exposure and Risk Assessment. 2013;**30**(3):534-540. DOI: 10.1080/19440049.2012.751630

[69] Nazarizadeh H, Pourreza J. Evaluation of three mycotoxin binders to prevent the adverse effects of aflatoxin B 1 in growing broilers. Journal of Applied Animal Research. 2019;**47**(1):135-139. DOI: 10.1080/09712119.2019.1584106

[70] Alsayyah A, ElMazoudy R, Al-Namshan M, Al-Jafary M, Alaqeel N. Chronic neurodegeneration by aflatoxin B1 depends on alterations of brain enzyme activity and immunoexpression of astrocyte in male rats. Ecotoxicology and Environmental Safety. 2019;**182**(February):109407

[71] Huang W, Cao Z, Yao Q, Ji Q, Zhang J, Li Y. Mitochondrial damage are involved in Aflatoxin B1-induced testicular damage and spermatogenesis disorder in mice. Science of the Total Environment. 2020;**701**:135077. DOI: 10.1016/j.scitotenv.2019.135077

[72] Agnew J. Market based solutions for addressing nutritional deficiencies: The case of Grameen Danone foods limited. [thesis]. University of Guelph; 2016. pp. 2-151

[73] Watson S, Gong YY, Routledge M. Interventions targeting child undernutrition in developing countries may be undermined by dietary exposure to aflatoxin. Critical Reviews in Food Science and Nutrition. 2017;**57**(9):1963-1975. DOI: 10.1080/10408398.2015.1040869

[74] Wen B, Bandsma RHJ. Understanding Pathways Underlying Inpatient Mortality of Children with Complicated Severe Malnutrition. Thesis Submitted to the Department of Nutrional Sciences, University of Toronto. 2022. p. 189. Available from: https://www.proquest.com/dissertations-theses/understanding-pathways-underlying-inpatient/docview/2644395293/se-2?accountid=266420A. http://link.periodicos.capes.gov.br/sfxlcl41?url_ver=Z39.88-2004&rft_val_fmt=info:ofi/fmt:kev:mtx:dissertation&genre=disser

[75] Raj J, Vasiljević M, Tassis P, Farkaš H, Bošnjak-Neumüller J, Männer K. Effects of a modified clinoptilolite zeolite on growth performance, health status and detoxification of aflatoxin B1 and ochratoxin A in male broiler chickens. British Poultry Science. 2021;**62**(4):601-610. DOI: 10.1080/00071668.2021.1891522

[76] Michael H, Amimo JO, Rajashekara G, Saif LJ, Vlasova AN. Mechanisms of Kwashiorkor- Associated immune suppression : Insights from human, mouse, and pig studies. Frontier in Immunology. 2022;**13**(May):1-19. DOI: 10.3389/fimmu.2022.826268

Chapter 4

Aflatoxins: A Postharvest Associated Challenge and Mitigation Opportunities

Anup Ramdas Kodape, Ashika Raveendran and Chikkarasanahalli Shivegowda Vivek Babu

Abstract

In agriculture, Aflatoxins are of major concern as they affect the nutrient quality of crops like Groundnut, Maize, and Coffee which are global economic commodities. Aflatoxin-contaminated products cause substantial financial losses and significant health problems in living beings. Aspergillus produces aflatoxins during environmental stress conditions. The International Agency for Research in Cancer (IARC) conducted studies on aflatoxins and found that Aflatoxin B1 (AFB1), Aflatoxin B2 (AFB2), Aflatoxin G1 (AFG1) and Aflatoxin G2 (AFG2) can cause cancer in both humans and animals and are classified into the Group 1 category of chemical hazards for potentiation mutagens. In India, the Food Corporation of India (FCI) monitors Aflatoxin levels in food and feeds. Aflatoxin contamination reduces the quality of groundnuts, maize, and coffee, affecting their exports. Consumption of aflatoxins contaminated feed induces liver cancer, immune suppressions, shunted growth, and in higher amounts, causes death. The current review provides information based on previous studies and newly adapted guidelines and methods showing the impact of aflatoxins on crops such as groundnut, coffee, and maize. The use of artificial intelligence to detect aflatoxin and mitigation opportunities using technologies such as Aflasafe, Aflaguard, hermetic bags, and Purdue Improved Crop Storage (PICS).

Keywords: aspergillus, aflatoxin, groundnuts, maize, coffee, biological control, artificial intelligence

1. Introduction

A new disease was identified with unknown characteristics in England during the 1950s and 1960s, which increased turkey mortality. Later, aflatoxin was recognized in 1960 in England as a causative agent of the mysterious Turkey 'X' disease that causes excessive mortality in the poults of Turkey (**Table 1**) [1–5]. The term aflatoxin (*Aspergillus flavus* toxin) was coined for this toxic agent [2]. Aflatoxins are low molecular weight and extremely toxic compounds. These are classified as the largest group of mycotoxins. The mold that includes the species of *Aspergillus* and *Penicillium* accounts for the spoilage of stored grains. Fungi under extreme

Year	Findings
1960	Outbreak of Turkey 'X' disease in England
	Aflatoxin discovery
1961	Identified *Aspergillus flavus* associated with toxicity of groundnuts
1962	Studies conducted on physicochemical properties of aflatoxins
	Aflatoxin B and G identified in TLC analysis
	Isolation and synthesis of crystalline aflatoxins
1963	Aflatoxin B2, G1, and G2 were identified and chemically characterized as
	Difurocoumarin derivatives
1965	FDA approved the first regulation on aflatoxins 30 μg/kg
1966	Milk toxins were designated as AFM1 and AFM2
	AFM1 was detected in Milk, Urine, Kidney, and liver
1967	Chemical synthesis of Aflatoxin B1
1969	FDA approved new limits for aflatoxins 20 μg/kg
1972	First IARC evaluation to detect the possible relationship between aflatoxins and liver Cancer in Humans
1974	The first outbreak of Aflatoxins affecting humans (106 deaths)
1975	IARC confirmed the carcinogenicity of Aflatoxins
1977	FDA approved new limits for aflatoxins AFM1 0.5 μg/kg
	DNA adducts of Aflatoxin B1 were identified
1981	DNA adducts of Aflatoxin B1 were identified in Urine
1987	IARC classified Aflatoxin in Group 1 as carcinogens
1991	Point mutation was identified on Codon 249 of the p53 gene
1992–1993	IARC confirmed Aflatoxin B1 as Group 1 carcinogen
1992	AFB1 and Liver cancer are linked was identified
1996	Aflatoxins producing fungi were detected in Grains by PCR analysis
2001	Establishment of Aflatoxin legal limit commission regulation (EC) no. 466/2001
2003	New terms of Aflatoxin legal limit commission regulation (EC) no. 2174/2003 for specific types of species
2004	An outbreak of aflatoxicosis in Kenya by consuming contaminated
2006	New regulations of Aflatoxin legal limit commission regulation (EC)
	no. 401/2006 for the limits of aflatoxins in foodstuffs
2012	Due to climatic conditions, cereals were affected, and a potential increase in aflatoxin B1 in the EU was observed
	IARC identified AFB1, AFB2, AFG1, and AFG2 are highly carcinogenic and are classified as Group 1 carcinogens
2014–2019	Neonatal exposure and Aflatoxin traces were found in the Umbilical cord (Nepal and Bangladesh)
2019	Around 25 Species of Aflatoxin-producing fungi were identified in sections Flavi, Nidulantes and Ochraceorosei

Year	Findings
2020	From section Flavi- A. texensis, *A. agricola* and *A. toxicus* are able for production of aflatoxins
2021	Aflatoxins Poisoning in Dogs (US) by consuming contaminated feed
Adopted and modified from Refs. [1–4].	

Table 1.
Timeline for Aflatoxin (1960–2021).

stress and inadequate maintenance, such as low nitrogen content, temperature, and drought, enhance aflatoxin accumulation in *Aspergillus spp*. *A. flavus* contaminates oilseed, stored grains, and coffee in pre and postharvest conditions. Globally, FAO (The Food and Agricultural Organization of United Nations) has provided regulations on mycotoxin content in both food and feeds, and FDA (Food and Drug Administration) has assigned specific limits for aflatoxins for human consumption, i.e., 20 ppb (parts per billion) and 0.5 ppb in food and dairy products respectively. A person infected with the hepatitis B virus who ingests aflatoxin-contaminated food has a higher risk of developing hepatic cancer [6]. European Union (EU) has specified stringent standards of value 4 ppb for aflatoxins. Several approaches have been explored to examine Aflatoxins present in foods such as TLC, HPLC, ELISA, LC-MS/MS, and others. HPLC, combined with fluorescence detection, is an analytical method widely used for detecting aflatoxins in different food samples (**Table 2**).

1.1 Aflatoxins and stored grains

1.1.1 Groundnut

Groundnut is a leading oil production crop and a highly traded commodity. China ranks first for groundnut production globally with 17.57 million metric tons (MMT) of quantity. India produces 6.93 MMT, Nigeria, 4.45MMT, Sudan 2.83 MMT, and US 2.49MT. Furthermore, groundnut production will be 81.56 MMT in 2020–2022. The estimated groundnut production in 2021–2022 will be 82.54 MMT. The fungi, namely *Aspergillus flavus* and *Aspergillus parasiticus* that produce aflatoxins, contaminate the field, resulting in significant loss of groundnut production. Due to this, the yield is reduced by 13–59%, particularly during warm and humid conditions. Pests account for an estimated 39% of all losses, leading to increased economic loss. Drought is yet another contributor to the decline in groundnut production. These conditions favor the growth of opportunistic molds, which enhances field contamination higher and loss of yield. An estimated 20–30% of groundnut loss occurs due to damaged pods during the postharvest. This merely relies on the techniques used for post-harvesting and the soil's moisture content. Insect activity in storage conditions increases the chances of contamination up to 6–10%. In Gujrat, groundnut is harvested during June and October twice a year. In both cases, there is a high risk of experiencing rain during drying harvested crops which causes heavy damage to a pod. Around 50% turned black due to mold infections. In such conditions, molds produce aflatoxins, which reduces seeds' quality and market value (**Figure 1**).

S. No.	Mycotoxins	Major producing fungi	Major substrates in nature	US FDA µg/Kg	EU µg/Kg	FSSAI µg/Kg	IARC No.*
1	Alternaria (AM) Mycotoxins	*Alternaria alternata*	Cereal grains, tomato, animal feeds	—	—	15	—
2	Aflatoxin (AF) B1	*Aspergillus flavus*	Peanuts, corn, cottonseed, cereals	20	2–12 for AFB1 4–15 Total AF	15	1*
3	Other aflatoxins	*Aspergillus parasiticus*	Walnuts	20 for total	4–15 total	15	1*
4	Citrinin (CT)	*Penicillium citrinum*	Barley, corn, rice, walnuts	—	—	—	2B*
5	Cyclopiazonic acid (CPA)	*Aspergillus flavus, P. cyclopium*	Peanuts, corn, cheese	—	—	—	—
6	Deoxynivalenol (DON)	*Fusarium graminearum*	Wheat, corn	1000	200–50	1000	3*
7	Cyclochloronitine (CC)	*P. islandicum*	Rice	—	—	—	—
8	Fumonisins (FM)	*F. moniliforme*	Corn, sorghum	2000–4000	200–4000	—	2B*
9	Luteoskyrin (LT)	*P. islandicum, P.rugulosum*	Rice, sorghum	—	—	—	—
10	Moniliformin (MN)	*F. moniliforme, A.ochraceus*	Corn, Barley, cereals, feeds, maize, oats, rice	—	—	—	—
11	Ochratoxin A (OTA)	*A. verrucosum*	Rice, wheat	not set	02–10	20	2B*
12	Patulin (PT)	*P.patulum, P.urticae, A.clavatus*	Wheat, apple, beans	50	10–50	50	3*
12	Penicillic acid (PA)	*Aspergillus ochraseus*	Foodstuff, corn	—	—	—	—
14	Penitrem A (PNT)	*P.palitance*	Barley, corn	—	—	—	—
15	Roquefortine (RQF)	*P.roqueforti*	Cheese	—	—	—	—
16	Rubratoxin B (RB)	*P.rubrum, P.purpurogenum*	Corn. Soyabean	—	—	—	—
17	Sterigmatocystin (ST)	*Aspergillus versicolor, A. nidulance*	Corn, grains, cheese	—	—	—	—

DOI: http://dx.doi.org/10.5772/intechopen.106333

18	T-2 Toxin	*F.sporotrichioides*	Corn, feeds, hay	15	25–1000	—	3*
19	12–13, Epoxy trichothecenes other than T-2 and DON	*F.nivale*	Corn, feeds, hay, peanuts, rice	15	25–1000	—	3*
20	Zearalenone (ZE)	*F. graminerium*	Cereals, corn, feeds, rice	—	20–100	—	3*

Adopted and modified from Refs. [7–9].
NOT SET = —.

Table 2.
Mycotoxins and their respective substrates. (IARC defines 1 for carcinogenicity to humans; 2B as Possible carcinogenic; 3 as not classified as a carcinogen to humans).

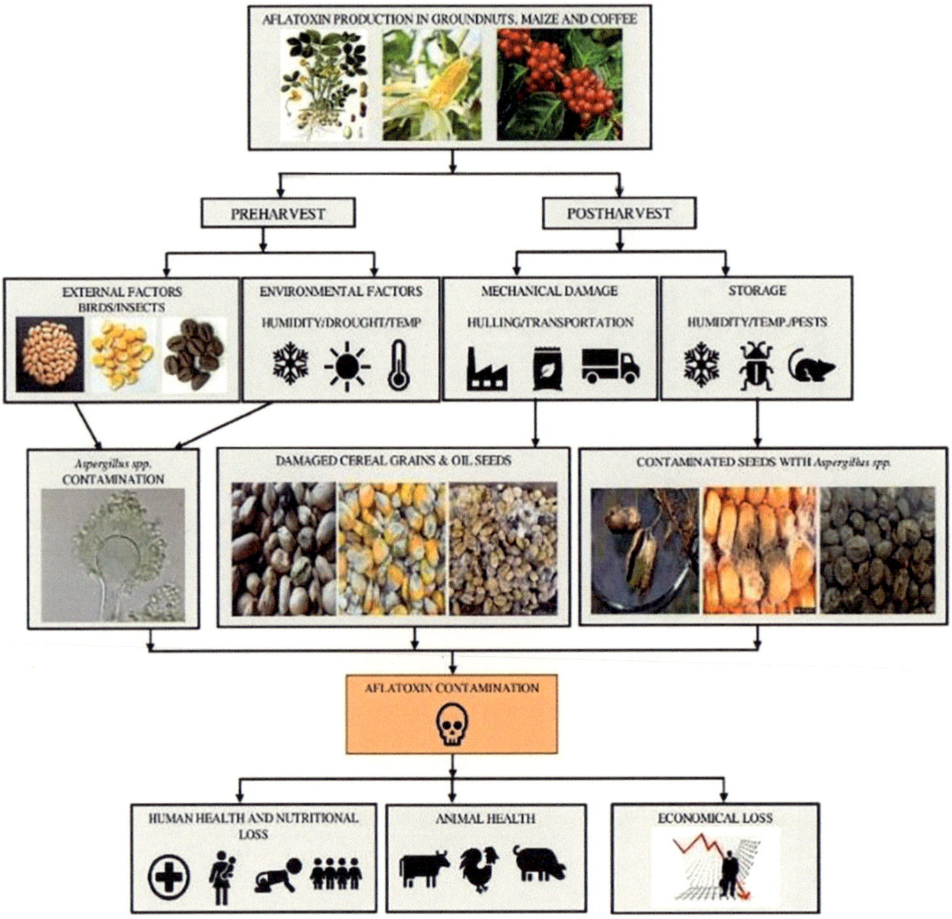

Figure 1.
Effects of Aflatoxin contamination in Groundnut, Maize, and Coffee.

1.1.2 Maize

The US produces a high quantity of maize, around 360.252 MMT of maize/year; after that, China produces 260.67 MMT, Brazil 109 MMT, EU 63.6 MMT, Argentina 47.5 MMT, Ukraine 29.5 MMT, India 28.5 MMT, Mexico 28 MMT. In 2021, the United States Department of Agriculture (USDA) estimated a world corn production in 2020–2021 to be 1133.89 MMT compared to 2019–2020. The 1133.89 MMT shows a surge of 1.57% in corn production around the globe. In India, 50%-60% of the harvested crops are stored by traditional methods in households and fields for consumption during scarcity. However, poor management causes 40%–45% damage to stored maize. In maize, contamination appears because of unexpected weather conditions, and insect infestation causes 0.2–11.8% weight loss [10]. During corn filling, birds eat kernels and damage the plant, which causes fungal spores deposition and eventually infects the plant and imparts increased agricultural losses. *A. flavus* is a saprotrophic and opportunistic parasitic fungus that causes severe loss of crops in the field. The average loss by mycotoxins and pests per year is around 20%–30% in maize due to inappropriate practices in agriculture and improper storage management, accounting for 5%–7% loss (**Figure 1**) [11].

1.1.3 Coffee

Coffee is a global commodity consumed daily by millions of people. It is a highly traded commodity worldwide. Asia will be the third-largest coffee producer during 2019–2020. Indian coffee accounts for 3.14% of global coffee production, i.e., approximately 299,300 MT of coffee production. In contrast, the total export was US $490.59 Million between April–November 2019 and 298000MT of coffee production, approximately US $459.87 million in April–November 2020. There is an increased risk of infection by molds during harvest and storage by the fungi, including *Aspergillus flavus*, *Aspergillus paraciticus*, *Penicillium*, etc. [12]. These molds grow in humid and moist environments. The temperature also influences their growth. Before storage, coffee beans are dried until the moisture level reaches 11%–12%. The semi-dry method is a combination of both dry and wet methods. Recent studies found that at 10% humidity, molds can produce 4.387 μg/g of aflatoxin. In 25% humidity, they produce 10.436 μg/g of aflatoxin. In 45% humidity of storage, the coffee beans are highly susceptible to Aflatoxins and produce 4.604 μg/g of aflatoxin resulting in quality loss of beans (**Figure 1**).

1.2 Aflatoxin outbreaks

In India, the disease was initially recognized in 1966 in chicks, leading to thousands of chicks' mortality. The cause of mortality was recognized by the Government poultry breeding unit in Bangalore. The first aflatoxin poisoning outbreak in India in 1974 caused 106 deaths by ingesting contaminated maize [13]. Besides this, in 1982, the Chittoor, a district in Andhra Pradesh, reported a loss of heavy chick mortality as a cause of aflatoxicosis. Due to this, poultry farms remained shut during this period. To combat this, in 1985, egg production was discontinued to reduce loss during outbreaks of aflatoxicosis in the Warangal district of Andhra Pradesh. In the Mysore district of Karnataka, the first reports of aflatoxicosis were in 1966. This outbreak resulted in the mortality of 2219 chick's poultry farms. Similarly, South Canara and Ranga-Reddi districts of Andhra Pradesh recorded 200,000 chickens dying due to aflatoxin poisoning [14].

In the study conducted in 1993 by the International Agency for Research in Cancer (IARC), it was concluded that sufficient data is available for trials in animals for the AFM1 carcinogenicity. However, the information on AFM1 in humans is inadequate [14]. Researchers suggest that seasonal variations in aflatoxin exposure could be correlated with food availability [15]. Humans can experience various symptoms due to Aflatoxins depending on their health conditions, age factors, duration of infection, and level of contamination in their body. Prolonged aflatoxin consumption in humans can result in hepatic cancer. They are much more susceptible to acquiring hepatitis B and cause initial stages of jaundice [6]. India has 40 million active hepatitis B virus (HBV) carriers, approximately 10.15% of the global population. Around 15–40% of infected patients develop symptoms like cirrhosis, liver failure, and hepatic carcinoma [16]. The same symptoms are observed in aflatoxicosis, so it may be concluded that both Aflatoxin and HBV are closely associated. Coffee is also consumed by billions of people worldwide. This crop is vulnerable to aflatoxin and may result in a pandemic if the toxin levels are not controlled. It leads to adverse human health effects. In India, 86 million people live in extreme poverty, accounting for approximately 6% of the country's total population (May 2021), whose access to low-quality foods and unhygienic environments increases the vulnerability of rural communities as a whole perfect hotspot for such toxicants. In such instances, food protection and policies for aflatoxin control must be established and regularly monitored in these regions. The World economic forum conducted a study that states that India may suffer from aflatoxicosis in the future since they cannot afford a portion of good quality food and are still coping with scarcity and consuming contaminated food.

1.3 Food safety governing bodies and the impact of aflatoxins on the food chain

Food Corporation of India (FCI) was set up under the Food corporation act 1964 to manage food policies for farmers. They also maintain satisfactory operational Safety stock of food grains for the nation's safety. Food Safety and Standards Authority of India (FSSAI) was established under the Food safety and standard act 2006, a law regulating food products and enforcing food safety standards in India. FSSAI promotes and regulates public health through regulations and regular food safety management in India. On 19 August 2020, FSSAI notified a publication that a first amendment regulation limited the various contaminants, including metals, aflatoxins, and mycotoxins. In a new regulation by governing bodies, aflatoxin's permissible value for grains and food products is 10 μg/kg.

After ingesting aflatoxin-contaminated food products, experience abdominal pain, vomiting, pulmonary edema, liver necrosis, extensive proliferation of bile duct, and fat infiltrations; few studies on aflatoxins stated that it causes growth suppression. It is also reported that Aflatoxins cause carcinogenic activity in animal models, confirming their carcinogenic potency. According to the studies conducted by Wogan et al. [17], rats are prone to toxins. It was observed that the clinical administration of rats with doses of 1, 5, 15, 50, 100 ppb could induce tumors in the liver, implying that even a microgram of aflatoxin can induce cancer. Among the 14 naturally occurring aflatoxins, AFB1, AFB2, AFG1 and AFG2 are potentially carcinogenic and can damage the coffee beans in storage. AFB1 is categorized as extremely carcinogenic and is added to the group 1 category by IARC. The remaining aflatoxins are categorized as a possible carcinogen that belongs to group 2B because of their toxicity and carcinogenicity [18]. In a study on coffee beans, 20–30% of *Aspergillus flavus* are widely isolated that can produce B type of aflatoxin. *Aspergillus parasiticus* produces both AFB and AFG in coffee beans. The toxic nature of the AFG family is lower than the AFB family [19].

Aflatoxins are usually identified based on the fluorescence they emit in UV light. Fluorescence blue (B) series toxins are represented as the fusion of cyclopentane ring with lactone ring of coumarins (**Table 3**), and green fluorescence (G) series toxin contains fused lactone rings. AFB2 and AFG2 remain non-toxic unless the metabolic oxidization internally by humans and animals forms AFB1 and AFG1. These forms of aflatoxins (AFB1 and AFG1) possess unsaturated bonds at the 8–9 position of the terminal furan ring. The epoxidation at this position, catalyzed by P450 monooxygenase, results in the generation of epoxide, which can further react with DNA adduct, i.e., Aflatoxin N7 guanine, which is critical for its carcinogenic potency. Aflatoxin M1 (AFM1) and Aflatoxin M2 (AFM2) are hydroxylated forms of AFB1 and AFB2 in cattle milk by consuming contaminated feeds. Several studies suggest the correlation between aflatoxin and point mutation. This mutation occurs at a specific location, i.e., at the third base of codon 249 in the p^{53} gene, resulting in the transversion of guanine to thymidine, which was observed in liver cancer in African patients [20].

In contrast, few studies reveal that aflatoxins carcinogenicity is independent of p^{53} gene mutations [21]. Structure elucidation of AFB1was identified in early 1963,

S. No	Aflatoxins	Aflatoxin producing fungi
Difuranocoumarins series		
1	AFB1	*A. flavus, A. arachidicola, A. bombycis, A. nomius, A. rambelli, A. ochraceoroseus.*
2	AFB2	*A. nomius, A. parasiticus, A. flavus, A. arachificola, A. minisclerotigenes*
3	AFB2A	*A. flavus*
4	AFM1	*A. flavus, A. parasiticus*
5	AFM2	Metabolite of AFB2
6	AFM2A	Metabolite of AFM1
7	AFLATOXICOL	*A. flavus,* Metabolite of AFB1
8	AFLATOXICOL M1	*Metabolites of AFM1*
Difuranocoumarolactone series		
9	AFG1	*A. flavus, A. arachidicola, A. minisclerotigenes, A. nomius, A. parasiticus*
10	AFG2	*A. flavus, A. arachidicola, A. minisclerotigenes, A. nomius, A. parasiticus*
11	AFG2A	Metabolite of AFG2
12	AFGM1	*A. flavus*
13	AFGM2	Metabolite of AFG2
14	AFGM2A	Metabolite of AFGM2
15	PARASITICOL (P)	*A. flavus*
16	AFLATREM	*A. flavus, A. minisclerotigenes*
17	ASPERTOXIN	*A. flavus*
18	AFQ1	The major metabolite of AFB1

Table 3.
Aflatoxin-producing fungi and aflatoxin derivatives depending on the Difurocoumarin and Difurocoumarolactone series.

further validated by its total biosynthesis [22]. Foods with carbohydrate and lipid content are more susceptive to aflatoxin contamination. Once produced, they are highly stable and heat resistant. Therefore, removing aflatoxin is tedious and not eliminated by heat treatment. AFB1 is a highly heat-stable form of aflatoxin [23].

1.4 Aflatoxins in groundnut

Groundnuts *(Arachis hypogaea L.)* are extensively grown in semi-arid regions worldwide. It is produced and supplied in over a 100 nations to aid the global demand. Among the Asian continents, China is a massive cultivar. India contributes 65% of the groundnuts produced; the US and the African countries (26%) also cultivate groundnuts. Groundnuts are also termed peanuts, earthnuts, goobers, and monkey nuts. Globally, groundnuts are the 4th most traded among the oil seeds. Groundnuts are rich in proteins (20–50%), fats (40–50%), carbohydrates (10–20%) and soil content of around 33.6–54.95%. Groundnuts are safe to be consumed directly as raw or can be roasted and boiled.

Groundnuts are estimated to be approximately 95% of production in developing countries. Nevertheless, they are contaminated with aflatoxins and are impossible to be traded globally [24]. Aflatoxin contamination is a severe problem for groundnuts. These contaminations can arise during pre and postharvest periods, extreme weather, increased drought, or excessive precipitation. These conditions lead to increased humidity surrounding the kernels, resulting in groundnut pod infection, eventually affecting stored kernels. The ideal conditions that accelerate aflatoxins in groundnuts are high temperature (up to 45°C) and humidity (65–90%). Infestations by rodents, insect activity and inadequate storage management are the secondary causes that enhance the severity of contamination. Groundnut is an economically important crop. Poor management while cultivating and harvesting can cause considerable loss of cultivation and increase the economic burden. Aflatoxins are colorless, odorless, and flavorless, making these compounds untraceable. Both humans and animals can unintentionally consume the contaminated foods.

Aflatoxins are accountable for the contamination of many economically important cash crops. Many genetically modified species of groundnuts have been developed to address this issue. Planting the crop varieties resistant to aflatoxin-producing fungal species can be a cost-effective way to decrease the infections and eventually reduce the level of aflatoxin in groundnut. Aflatoxins are the group of mycotoxins [7] closely related to groundnuts as it has all the essential components for fungal growth. Due to contamination, most groundnuts are not exported to the international market due to strict guidelines about aflatoxin. Above the permissive limit, the food commodity is neither restricted for trade in the market nor used for other purposes. Since the groundnuts are not being used causes an economic loss. In temperate countries such as India and Africa, it is most likely to get contaminated with soil-borne fungal infections, as groundnuts are in direct exposure to the soil, which elevates the risk of getting infected in changed environmental conditions, eventually causing infestation on pods and plants. *Aspergillus flavus* and *Aspergillus parasiticus* invade groundnuts while harvesting, storage, and processing. These fungi infect the plant, reducing its yield, and produce aflatoxins in seeds. At the same time, if harvested groundnuts are kept in the field for a longer duration without proper management, there is a high risk of pods getting infected with many opportunistic aflatoxin-producing fungi. The insect activity also damages a kernel and results in gaps in the pods. From these gaps, fungi can enter the seeds, which remain inactive until the conditions are favorable for the growth and production of aflatoxins [25, 26].

Preharvest management of groundnuts includes several measures to avoid fungal infection, including cultivating resistant varieties, irrigation, managing insect activity, and crop rotation. These practices can decrease the level of fungal infestation in groundnut. Resistant varieties are not entirely immune to *Aspergillus spp.* However, it can be moderately resistant, which helps reduce aflatoxin-causing fungal growth. Irrigation practices aid in decreasing the temperature of the field as the fungus produces aflatoxins in higher temperatures. It is recommended that regular field irrigation can be beneficial for contamination and the proper management of plant pathogens. Irrigation can relieve drought stress and maintain the temperature of the soil [27]. During the initial stages of crop development, insect activity is a serious concern as it could damage plant parts. Insects also act as carriers of fungal spores from an infected plant to a non-infected plant and transfer the spores through minor incisions. Hence, insects are considered the primary cause of infections in plants. Its proper management in reducing the infections on crops is substantial. Insects including mites, beetles, grasshoppers, and thrips damage peanut kernels and make them more prone to infection by the *Aspergillus spp*. that results in the production of Aflatoxins in seeds.

Similarly, crop rotation is favorable for reducing fungal infections in groundnuts as aflatoxin-producing fungi are soil-borne. Using the non-host plant is an effective strategy for reducing the contamination level for subsequent harvest. Selection of the appropriate crop is crucial because if both plants are susceptible to the same fungi, it can be infectious to both the plants, contaminating the entire field in much more significant quantities and causing inconvenience for market export after the harvest [28].

Postharvest management includes steps after the crops have been harvested from the field. Groundnuts are adequately cleaned and dried until the seed's moisture content reaches 7%. It is crucial for storage since high moisture content in kernels can promote fungal activity leading to aflatoxin production in seeds. Storage spaces must be cleaned thoroughly before storage to avoid fungal and insect infestations. After the drying process, the kernels were transferred to storage rooms and kept for nearly 1 year at 25–27°C [29]. Insects can infect groundnuts during storage but can be managed with chemical pesticides. There is a higher risk of seed damage during transportation which the proper management of transport services can prevent. Recently, newer packing materials have been developed to protect groundnut against fungal infections. Infections can also be decreased by segregating infected and non-infected seeds. Although this is a laborious process, it effectively reduces the aflatoxin level. After extraction of healthy pods, the damaged pods must be immediately incinerated as many cultivars adulterate them with healthy pods for for-profit and endangering the lives of both humans and animals. Altered seeds are restricted from the international market due to the aflatoxin regulations. However, these are sold and utilized at the local markets at much lower prices. Government bodies should regularly monitor these practices to avoid aflatoxin contamination (**Figure 1**).

1.4.1 Phytochemical composition of groundnuts

Groundnuts are rich in nutritional value with high phytochemical components to prepare oils and animal feeds. The phytochemical analysis of groundnut seeds reveals the following compounds; tannins (822 ± 3.78 mg/100gm), saponins (438 ± 2.12 mg/100gm), nitrogen (1.33 ± 0.03 mg/100gm), phenolic acids (218.2.11 mg/100gm), phytic acid (572 ± 4.37 mg/100gm), flavonoids like catechins, epicatechins, apigenin, luteolin and phosphorus (700 ± 3.62 mg/100gm) [30]. Flavonoids have been shown to protect against heart diseases. It inhibits the oxidation of low-density lipoproteins and cholesterol, reducing the formation and circulation of free radicals in the body [31]. Recent researchers have identified a compound phytosterol β-sitosterol (SIT) in groundnut seeds, oils, and flour. This compound has been protective against different types of cancer such as Colon, Prostate and Breast cancers by blocking cholesterol absorption [32].

1.5 Aflatoxins in maize

Maize is an essential and staple agricultural crop that is consumed worldwide. In most regions of the world, maize is infected with aflatoxins, especially in tropical and subtropical areas. In terms of production, consumption, and revenue, maize is an essential commodity worldwide. Several countries do not impose safety standards on maize as they lack proper infrastructures, sampling protocols, and qualified personnel to monitor the standards. Due to high aflatoxin poisoning, more than a 100 countries have set specific limits for aflatoxin tolerance levels. Maize is the most traded food among cereal grains and significantly supports the world economy. However, the contaminations are the concerns that affect the quality of maize, lowering the market price that primarily impacts the underdeveloped countries, affecting the country's economic progress. The FDA and EU have issued guidelines for aflatoxins, which most countries accept [33, 34]. Many farmers continue using local varieties of maize. They have poor agricultural practices while farming, leading to plant infections and maize being contaminated with fungal spores [24]. When there are unfavorable weather conditions, the fungus produces aflatoxins and contaminates the maize.

Regions with high humidity increase the possibility of maize infection with aflatoxin-producing fungi such as *A. flavus* and *A. parasiticus.* Apart from these fungi, a section of Flavi, consisting of more than 18 fungi, can produce aflatoxins. To avoid infections from the aflatoxin-producing fungi, infected maize should be predisposed during its development. During maturation, the maize is more vulnerable to diseases as many bugs, insects, mites, beetles, and grasshoppers carry fungal spores on their body. When it attacks the plant, it gets damaged and injured. Fungal spores enter the plant through these incisions and habitat the plant until favorable conditions for growth. During adverse drought and elevated temperatures, fungi produce aflatoxins in response to environmental stimuli. Genetically modified species of maize can be a solution for decreasing contamination, but this technique is moderately effective. Another approach is that maize inhabits various atoxigenic fungi that may act as biocontrol agents to cope with aflatoxin contamination [35, 36].

Most farmers cultivate maize for self-consumption and store it in houses with less or no management, increasing the risk of contamination to a greater extent. Consumption of contaminated maize can cause stunted growth, immune suppression, cirrhosis and liver cancer. Safety regulations are followed in the global market to protect and safeguard human and animal health. However, in most developing countries, even with many regulations on aflatoxins, individuals tend to consume contaminated maize that has not been subjected to regulatory checks, which is a significant concern. Consumers should be well informed of the consequences of aflatoxin contamination, and specific awareness meetings should be organized to limit the aflatoxin level in food [24].

Aflatoxins that contaminate maize and its products can be of significant health concern to commercial and substantial farming. According to the FAO, globally, most of the cereal grains in the United States are affected by mycotoxin-producing fungi, increasing the economy's loss [34]. In the US, contamination of aflatoxin is less. However, animal feeds were often recalled due to higher levels of aflatoxin content [37]. Contaminated maize has been least recommended for food and feed consumption. To avoid losses, the contaminated maize, which contains high aflatoxin levels, is transferred to industries to be utilized as feed products that increase animal health risks. Low levels of aflatoxin-contaminated food that are regularly fed can induce liver cancer [38]. Animals express symptoms such as vomiting, feed refusal, weight loss, infertility, and impaired organ functions. Good agricultural management comprises all the steps from plantation to harvest and postharvest handling. The effective practices that help reduce the infections of opportunistic fungi use of Aflatoxin resistant plant varieties, irrigation, use of fungicides and insecticides, sorting, the safe disposal of the infected plant, moisture control measures, for instance, solar drying, trap drying, and improved storage conditions are effective practices that reduce the chances of the crop getting contaminated with fungi producing aflatoxins. The allowed limit of aflatoxins in maize for humans is 20 ppb, and for animals, it is

300 ppb. According to Nyandieka et al. [39], maize crops placed in a sealed container for 1–2 weeks, applied with ammoniation gas can decrease the aflatoxin level by 90%.

Similarly, Whitlow's studies show that to prevent the hazardous effects of aflatoxins on animals. Binding agents can be used in animal feeds to neutralize up to 90% of the aflatoxins from maize while processing [40]. Sorting good and contaminated maize, winnowing, washing, and crushing, combined with dehulling, effectively removes mycotoxins in maize grains. Maize can also be contaminated with other classes of mycotoxins, such as Fumonisins [7, 41].

1.5.1 Phytochemical composition of maize

Maize kernels are rich in polyphenolic components, phenolic acids, vitamins, carotenoids, polysaccharides, flavonoids, and sugars. Studies on maize silk flavonoids have shown antifatigue activity and reduced oxidative stress in mice. Even corn tassels are an excellent source of phytochemicals. In a study by Duangpapeng et al. [42], they found that 92.4% of antioxidants in a variety P4546 for DPPH (2,2-diphenyl-1-picryl-hydrazyl) [42]. Cornhusk consists of anthocyanins, and corn pollen contains phenolic compounds. Phytochemical analysis helps genetically modify the species to produce chemicals with better insecticidal activity and increased nutritional quality [27].

1.6 Aflatoxins in coffee

Coffee is consumed globally due to specific tastes and its various medicinal properties. Globally, coffee is a beverage widely consumed due to its health benefits, taste, aroma, pharmacological properties, and stimulant effects [43]. Various species are cultivated worldwide, but coffee arabica (60%) and robusta (40%) provide the global supply. It has been the second most exported commodity after petroleum and is crucial in supporting the economy. Wide coffee varieties are cultivated worldwide. Coffee Arabica and Coffee Robusta are major cultivars and dominate the coffee market. Coffee Arabica is mild and has more aroma than robusta.

In contrast, Robusta beans are dark with high caffeine content than coffee arabica. More than 80 species of coffee are grown in different regions of the world. In every society, coffee has historical, social, cultural, and economic value. Brazil has been the largest producer and exporter of raw coffee beans globally [44]. In 2018 2.13MT of coffee was exported, earning the US $ 5.14 Billion.

In India, coffee cultivation started in the 1600s. Beans were brought by Baba Budan from yamen and first grown in Chikmagalur district, Karnataka. Globally, India is the sixth-largest cultivar and trader of coffee. In the post-monsoon season (2020–2021), 342000MT of coffee has been harvested in India. The country's prominent coffee-producing regions are Karnataka, Kerala, Tamilnadu, Tripura, Nagaland, Assam Meghalaya, Manipur, Orissa, Andhra Pradesh, Arunachal Pradesh, And Chikhaldara [45]. In Chikmagalur, Karnataka, the average coffee production is 80300MT, 35800MT Coffee arabica, and 44500MT Coffee robusta. Around 250,000 cultivars are currently present in India, whose source of revenue is coffee cultivation. Indian coffee beans with production in different regions have different properties and qualities that can be attributed to several factors such as climatic conditions, soil topography, agricultural practices and harvest conditions that include both preharvest and post-harvest techniques (drying, wet process, storage, roasting, and grinding) [46]. Karnataka state contributes almost 71% of total coffee cultivation in

India, Kerala contributes 21%, Tamil Nadu 5%, and the remaining are small growers. The total coffee harvest consumed domestically in the country is 25–30%, and the remaining 70–75% is exported globally. Numerous factors directly or indirectly affect the cultivation in these regions where coffee arabica and Coffee robusta are produced.

Coffee has various metabolites, terpenes, phenols, and antioxidants. Caffeine is the principal constituent in coffee beans, a psychoactive compound. Regular coffee consumers are less likely to develop psychological disorders like Alzheimer's and Parkinson's. Due to environmental factors and infections caused by molds that produce aflatoxins, coffee cultivars face many issues. AFB1 has many secondary derivatives. The FDA sets specific limits safe intake of coffee and food products. AFB1 is highly resistant to heat, making it challenging to eliminate from the coffee beans. Aflatoxin endemics have resulted in the death of several people in India. Coffee is a major source of caffeine [47].

The caffeine content in coffee beans is a significant concern in the global market, as high caffeine tastes bitter. Caffeine, a psychoactive drug, can be beneficial if its intake is limited and harmful to health in higher doses. Besides health concerns, high caffeine is associated with coffee quality, eventually affecting the cost and consumer preference for coffee beans [48]. There are certain limits to caffeine content. For adults, 3–4 cups of coffee/day, i.e., 300 mg/day of caffeine, is considered moderate intake, and above 400 mg/day is the highest consumption limit [43, 49]. In 2006 Canadian health agencies set caffeine's upper limit as 450 mg/day, which is considered safe. In Australia, the recommended limit is 160 mg/day [49]. Caffeine can cause deleterious effects on health that include cardiovascular disturbance, miscarriage, restlessness, headache, excitement, muscular tension, increased blood sugar levels, sleep disturbance, increased pepsin secretion, and gastric acid secretions [49]. Caffeine can pass through the placenta. It is a stimulant; it increases the foetal heart rate and metabolic processes. Higher doses of caffeine elevate the risk of spontaneous abortion and impair fetus growth [50]. In adults, the moderate caffeine content in the blood can cause cardiovascular stimulatory effects and behavioral changes [51].

Coffee is rich in antioxidants. Several commercial companies market energy drinks with high caffeine content, and unknowingly, many consumers having a history of cardiovascular diseases ingest it, placing their lives at risk. In the Tromso heart study [52], it was observed that consumption of coffee could reduce the gamma-glutamyl transferase (GGT) level [53], and yet another study documented shows inverse relationships between coffee consumption and levels of aspartate aminotransferase (AST) and alanine aminotransferase (ALT) [54]. Besides caffeine, coffee has many aromatic compounds that give coffee its particular smell and taste. Its perception is dependent on the volatility of the compound present. Grosch studied many aromatic compounds in coffee. The study identified around 900 volatile compounds, but lesser than 20 compounds have been associated with coffee aroma. Consumption of coffee has beneficial effects on health and was found to have hepatoprotective effects. In 2015, Lui F. conducted a study on the consumption of coffee and found out that those who consume coffee have reduced incidences of cirrhosis compared to non-consumers of coffee (**Figure 1**) [55].

1.6.1 Phytochemical composition of coffee

Caffeine (1, 3, 7 trimethyl xanthine) is found in coffee beans, and apart from beans, it occurs in other plant parts [52, 56]. Caffeine is a psychoactive drug utilized by pharma companies to treat Alzheimer's and Parkinson's disease [57]. It has non-selective adverse effects on adenosine receptors, specifically at A1 and A2A positions. These receptors (A1 and A2A) are in a consistent reaction and only work in the presence of stimulatory G protein. A1 receptors affect the portion of the brain that controls the sleep and wake cycle, and the A2A receptor is present in the dopamine-rich areas of the brain. By forming heterodimers, A2A receptors coexist with dopamine D1 and D2. Chlorogenic acid (polyphenol) [52, 58] is primarily a phenolic ester of trans-cinnamic acid and quinic acid, also known as 5-o-caffeoylquinic acid [59]. It regulates glucose and lipid metabolism, cardiovascular diseases, cancer, and hepatic steatosis [60]. Also, few studies reported anti-diabetic, anti-carcinogenic [46], and anti-inflammatory activities.

Coffee beans have fat-soluble lipids such as kahweol and cafestol [52, 61]. These diterpenes originated from the isoprenoid metabolic pathway. An isoprenoid is a varied group of plant metabolites [62]. These diterpenes increase the blood cholesterol level in humans if consumed unfiltered. Post et al. [63] found that coffee brew consumption increases the cholesterol level [63]. In an experiment, bile acid mass production was measured on 24 hours basis with 8 hours of preincubated rats fed with cafestol, kahweol, and isokahweol mixture in a proportion of 48:47:5w/w, which resulted in a decline of bile production showing 91 ± 5% and 68 ± 3% inhibition [63]. Kahweol is highly unstable when purified. Thus, its properties are studied in combination. They are diterpenes with anti-cancerous properties. These diterpenes have been reported to act against AFB1 in humans. Also, these compounds can produce various biochemical processes that decrease the genotoxicity of cancer-causing agents such as DMBA, AFB1, BaP, and PhlP. The studies by IARC categorize coffee as non-carcinogenic for humans.

Several bioactive were isolated and identified from coffee leaves, including alkaloids, flavonoids, terpenoids, xanthonoids, phenolic acids and catechins, tannins, and sucrose [64]. Emura reported that the floral parts have aromatic nitrogenous compounds and phenylethane derivatives. In fruits, caffeine and tannins are present, which have antioxidant properties. Green beans of coffee consist of 7–17% of lipids, phenolic, and chlorogenic acids. These compounds can inhibit oxidative damage by free radical scavenging in biosynthesis and improve CCl4-induced liver damage by inhibiting the CYPZE1 liver-inducing enzyme and forming free radicals. Coffee oil consists of various bioactive compounds, and it was found that these metabolites can cure diabetes type 2 conditions [43, 65], cancer [65], and inflammation [52]. According to Velazquez Pereda Mdel et al. [66], green coffee oil affects elastin, collagen, and glycosaminoglycan synthesis [67].

2. Biosynthesis of aflatoxins

In 1967, Birch first proposed that a polyketide pathway is required for aflatoxin production [68]. Aflatoxins have similar structures, which are dihydrofuran coumarin derivatives (**Table 3**) [69]. Biosynthesis of Aflatoxins is a long series of processes requiring a minimum of 30 genes grouped inside 75 bp gene clusters and regulated by specified transcription factors. In the early 1990s, molecular biologists studied aflatoxin biosynthesis. In 1992 first gene was identified, isolated and transcribed (nor 1 and ver 1); later, a complete gene clustered for aflatoxin biosynthesis was identified. Concerning sequencing, *A. flavus* and *A. parasiticus* have similar gene clusters. However, they vary in deletion, ranging from 0.8 kb (L strain) and 1.5 kb

(S strain) [70]. In the case of *A. flavus,* deletion extends from 5'end of *aflF, aflU* to whole 279 bp intrinsic loci, which prevents it from producing the Aflatoxin G1 (AFG1) and Aflatoxin G2 (AFG2). The DNA analysis of *A. flavus* and *A. parasiticus* shows a 96% affinity for the gene clusters. For the aflatoxin biosynthesis in *A. flavus,* there are 30 pathway genes involved, including the antisense gene (afl R), three sugar utilization genes, and ORF genes, all of which are clustered within the 80 kb DNA region. *A.parasiticus* has 25 pathway genes consisting of sugar utilization genes and ORF genes clustered within the 80 kb DNA region [69]. For Norsolorinic acid (NOR) synthesis, three transcription factors are involved, the *aflA* gene (Fatty acid synthase A), *aflB* gene (Fatty acid synthase B), and *aflC* gene (Polyketide synthase), which helps in Norsolorinic acid synthase (NorS) production [71]. NorS utilized in synthesizing hexanoyl primer by integrating with the molecules of malonyl CoA. Hexanoyl primer shifts towards β-ketoacyl synthase and attaches to malonyl CoA, forming Norsolorinic acid anthrone (NAA). In the presence of NAA oxidase, it turns into Norsolorinic acid. This step is a crucial metabolite for aflatoxin biosynthesis [72]. Next, the *aflD* gene (Reductase), a NOR 1'keto group, is reduced by ketoreductase to the AVN 1'hydroxyl group. Even if it has defined work, the mutant strain of the aflD gene does not always lead to the formation of AVN. The gene *aflG* encodes cytochrome P450 mono-oxygenase which catalyzes the breakdown of AVN on the 5'keto group, which then converts into a 5′ hydroxyl group of 5'Hydroxyaverantin (HAVN) in *A.parasiticus* [73]. The *aflH* gene (dehydrogenase) 5'hydroxyaverantin dehydrogenase help in the dehydrogenation of the 5'hydroxyl group of HAVN to the 5'oxide group of oxoaverantin (OAVN) [74]. *AflK* gene (OAVN Cyclase) catalyzes the hydration of 5'oxide of OAVN to form the 2′-5'Averufin (AVF). *aflV* gene encodes P450 oxidoreductase, which reduces the hydride groups from AVF, and the *aflI* gene encodes the function of an oxidoreductase. *aflW* gene encodes monooxygenase, which incorporates O2 atoms within 4′-5′ ketone groups of HAVN, producing Versiconal hemiacetal acetate (VHA). VHA acetate is stimulated by the *aflJ* gene (Esterase) enzyme, eradicating and converting it into Versiconal (VAL) [75]. Afterwards, the *aflK* gene encodes the cyclase enzyme, which helps catalyze the cyclodehydration of VAL and converts it into Versicolorin B (VERB). In this step, bisfuran ring closure has occurred. It acts as a final precursor for the aflatoxin biosynthetic pathway and is an important step. *AflL* gene (desaturase) converts the tetrahydrofuran ring to dihydrobisfuran in the presence of the enzyme cytochrome P450 monooxygenase. VERA is utilized for the formation of Demethylsterigmatocystin (DMST), *aflM(ver1), aflN(ver1), aflY(hypA) and aflX(ordA)* enzymes are needed to produce AFB1-AFG1 [76]. Similarly, for the AFB2-AFG2 biosynthetic pathway, VERB is utilized as a substrate, leading to Dihydro-Demethylsterigmatocystin (DHDMST). *aflO* gene encodes O-methyltransferase and helps convert the S-adenosylmethionine methyl group, DMST hydroxyl group, and synthesis of sterigmatocystin from DHDMST and DHSD based on the Aflatoxin biosynthetic pathway. *aflP* is another gene which encodes O-methyltransferase, suitable for substrates like sterigmatocystin but can catalyze DHST and DHOMST. *aflQ* gene encodes cytochrome P450 monooxygenase, which helps transform OMST into the Aflatoxin B1 (AFB1)/Aflatoxin G1 (AFG1). Yu suggested *aflQ* gene replicated in C-11 hydroxylation. In contrast, the keto tautomer 11 hydroxy of the OMST *aflL* gene might serve as an Oxygen (O2) source [77]. *aflM* demethylates a ring that works with cytochrome P450 as a final aflatoxin biosynthetic pathway. The *aflV* gene oxidizes the metabolites produced in the process, which are then utilized as a substrate for the formation of the final intermediate, which is then

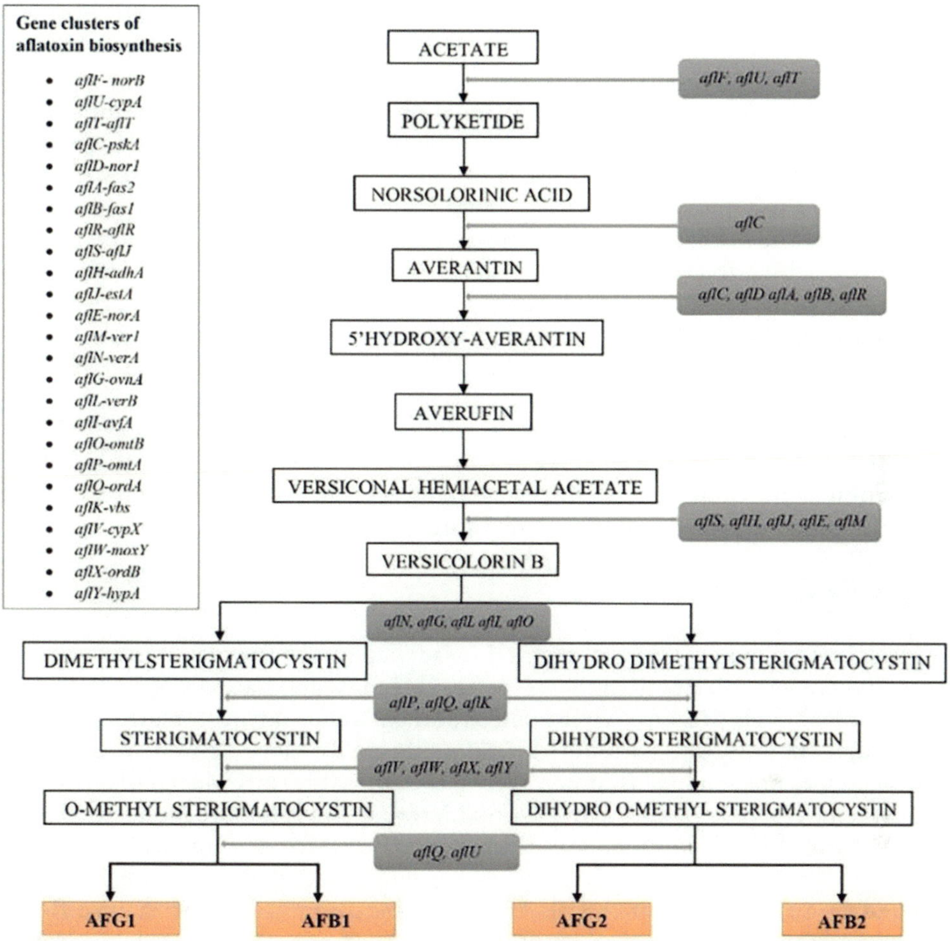

Figure 2.
Modified and adapted Flow diagram for Biosynthetic pathway of Aflatoxins [25, 77].

catalyzed by the *nadA* gene and the *aflF* gene. The product is obtained as an AFG1 [69, 78]. *aflU* encodes a reductase and cytochrome p450 monooxygenase, and the *nadA* gene helps catalyze the DHDMST to form an AFG2. So the *aflE(norA)* and *aflF(norB)* genes are suitable substrates for enhancing the activity for the production of AFG1 and AFG2 [69, 70] (**Figure 2**).

3. Prevention and management of Aflatoxin contamination

To detoxify and reduce aflatoxin levels in crops, it is crucial to intervene in both preharvest and postharvest processes. During pre-harvest, good agricultural practices, environmental factors, soil conditions, and certified fertilizers are the vital factors that help in plant development. The use of biological agents aids in reducing aflatoxin-producing fungi by eradicating them from the field. It is an effective preharvest strategy.

Postharvest techniques involve chemical methods, ammonification, the use of hydrated oxides, and biological agents. Oxidation, reduction, hydrolysis, and absorption have been performed in the chemical process [7]. Treatment with ammonia reduces aflatoxin to an untraceable level, but ammonia can be harmful to human health. Thus, European Union (EU) forbids treatment with bases for food intended for consumption by humans. Calcium hydroxide is used to the degenerate structure of aflatoxin AFB1 and reduce the toxicity. These chemicals can have harmful effects on food products and human health. Sorbent additions like silica, alumina, and aluminosilicates can bind to aflatoxins, minimizing the toxic effects. Sodium bisulfate can deprive Aflatoxins (AFB1) molecules in humans and animals on DNA reaction sites, thus decreasing the mutagenic potential of aflatoxin [7]. Another method for reducing aflatoxin includes epoxide hydrolase and glutathione-s-transferase [61]. It detoxifies the activated AFB1, glutathione conjugates with AFB1 8, 9 epoxides converted into glutathione aflatoxin conjugate and finally removed from the cell. CYP1A2 is effective in the hydroxylation of AFB1 to less potent AFM1, a poor substrate of epoxidation by the catalysis of cytoplasmic reductase enzyme, which converts AFB1 into AFQ1 that is excreted from the body by urination [61].

3.1 Aflasafe®

Aflasafe is a biological control method for managing the fungal strain of *Aspergillus flavus,* which contaminates food and feeds with aflatoxin. Aflatoxins are harmful metabolites produced in farms and storage rooms during stressful conditions such as high humidity and extreme heat. Afla safe is a developed strain of *Aspergillus flavus* that does not produce aflatoxin. When the Aflasafe is introduced in farming fields, it removes toxic strains with non-toxic strains. This phenomenon is known as competitive exclusion, as it increases competition between two strains of the same fungi [79]. Bandopadhyay and their research group have reported around 80% aflatoxin reduction in fields treated with Aflasafe stains compared to non-treated fields [27]. Aflasafe shows a promising result, particularly in crop fields and storage rooms. Even after the harvest, it does not allow the toxic strain of *Aspergillus flavus* to produce aflatoxins. This has long-term benefits, lowering the need for fungicides in storage rooms. For commercialization, farmers should utilize Aflasafe as it helps reduce contaminated crops and helps produce safe staple food [80]. Adopting Aflasafe can be beneficial for the reduction of contaminations in a staple food (maize), resulting in higher prices and a rise in the economy. Food safety levels can be maintained and stored for longer durations with proper management [27, 79].

The International Institute of Tropical Agriculture (IITA) has developed Aflasafe SN1 in a Nigerian laboratory according to the methodology adopted by Atehnkeng et al. 2014. Since this region is at a higher risk for aflatoxin contamination, trials were conducted to determine the efficacy of the Aflasafe SN1 in reducing aflatoxin contamination in oilseeds (Groundnut) from 2010 to 2013 results suggested reduced aflatoxin contamination. AG RESULTS Projects have promoted Aflasafe adoption [79].

3.2 Aflaguard®

Aflaguard has a solid brown appearance with a barley-like odor. Aflaguard is a biologically designed aflatoxin controlling agent which reduces *Aspergillus flavus* growth [81]. It consists of the non-toxigenic *Aspergillus flavus* strain (NRRL21882), which does not produce aflatoxin but can be competitive. Aflaguard is used in both corn and groundnut fields. The company recommends a quantity of 20 lb./acre which can be applied with the help of a tractor-mounted Grandy box or broadcast applications. Aflaguard should be applied to plants only after 40–80 days of a plantation. Aflaguard can be applied through the air with the same quantity, i.e., 20 lb./acre for groundnuts. In maize, Aflaguard GR can be applied during the V7 and R1 growth stages (the V7 stage refers to the growth period where seven visible leaf colors are present, and the R1 stage refers to the onset of silking) with the broadest application equipment. Precautions should be taken that all the cultivation and mechanical activities have been completed before the application of Aflaguard GR. The recommended limit of Aflaguard® GR is per season. Precautionary measures, such as PPE kits, must be used using Aflaguard® [82].

3.3 Hermetic bags

Grain pro® is a global company in concord, Massachusetts, established in 1992 and specialized in Ultrahermatic technologies for storage, transportation, and drying agricultural solutions. Grain pro company has many collaborations with various organizations worldwide, which help them develop a sustainable system for postharvest management. Grain pro products are Grain pro cocoon, Grain pro bags zipper, and Grain pro transafeliner. These developed products support chemical-free and organic. Hermetic bags has been utilized to dry, store, and transport agricultural commodities. It supports moisture-free, insects free and mold-free conditions. Grain pro bags helps in protecting the commodities against mold interactions, insecticidal activities, oxidation, and rancidity. These products contribute to keeping the food safe, preventing significant costs associated with pests, and manage mold during storage. Grain pro products used by farmers can help avoid food spoilage losses and maintain the quality of seeds in these bags [83].

3.4 Purdue improved crop storage (PICS)

PICS bags were developed by Purdue University in collaboration with private entrepreneurs and vendors. PICS bags are of 50 kg and 100 kg capacity and cost around $2USD-$4USD. PICS bags are high-density polyethene bags that are 80 μm in thickness. PICS comprises three bags; the inner bag is filled with grains and covered with another bag, the middle. Then these two bags are covered by a bag made from woven polypropylene. Woven bags are thick. Inner liners have less permeability for oxygen. The middle bag is tightly packed above the innermost bag and should surround without gaps. The outer woven bag is tied over those two bags. The advantage of PICS bags is that this method is devoid of fumigants and insecticide use. Thousands of smallholder farmers adopt PICS bags to store grains, showing promising results by reducing contamination levels and insecticidal activity. Farmers can utilize the same bags multiple times for a longer time. These bags can help achieve food security goals and preserve nutritional value. PICS bags helps in minimizing mold growth, management of insect pests, controlling mycotoxin accumulation, and postharvest loss [84].

3.5 Artificial intelligence (AI) and aflatoxin

Artificial intelligence is a program designed to develop intelligent machines that can work with higher accuracy. Artificial intelligence aids in understanding the processes that can predict and develop 3D structures of materials in scientific fields.

Pure scan AI is a newly developed technology that is a portable and easy-to-use device that can detect aflatoxins in groundnuts and maize via spectroscopic (UV) accessible scan technology integrated with Artificial Intelligence (https://purescanai.com) [85]. It is cost-effective and can identify contamination in less than 30 seconds, with an accuracy of 10 ppb. Results can be monitored on any device. The mechanism of this device is that cameras with filters capture an aflatoxin fluorescence. The captured images are processed through a program to detect the degree of fluorescence patterns, which helps predict the level of aflatoxin contamination in a sample. Pure scan AI is a startup company. The International Crops Research Institute for the SemiArid Tropics (ICRISAT) Hyderabad scientists Dr. Hari Sudini and Dr. Shrikanth Rupavatharam have collaboratively developed an Aflascan AI device to detect aflatoxin-contaminated groundnuts and maize with a 1 ppb accuracy. It is an integrated system of UV lights, and the results can be observed on any android device. This device costs around INR50000 (Indian Rupees) and per test INR8.

4. Discussion

Aflatoxin contamination is a significant cause of contamination on oilseeds (groundnuts), staple food (maize), and commodities (coffee). These food products are widely traded worldwide and are supplied for making food products for human and animal consumption. Due to improper management, fungi damage and contaminate the groundnut, maize, and coffee during their initial harvesting and storage conditions. Excessive drought and humidity increase the chances of infection. This is likely to increase if the crops are prone to insects, rodents, and birds attacking during the pre-harvest. The damages that occur in the crop pave the way for the opportunistic fungi *Aspergillus flavus* to penetrate the plant and stay dormant until favorable environmental conditions occur. Fungal spores can stay inactive for more extended periods. That is why, after postharvest, fungi are still attached to the harvested product. In storage rooms, deposited fungi grow and infest the whole batch of bags under optimum temperature and produce aflatoxins, which are harmful toxins for humans and animals.

Groundnut is the most traded oilseed which is cultivated worldwide. Just after removing the oils from seeds, the remaining residues of seeds are utilized to make animal feeds. All the parts of the seeds are ultimately used, making it a perfect food. Groundnuts are rich in proteins and are a valuable crop. It is susceptible to fungal infections, and *Aspergillus* is a significant contaminant that produces aflatoxins in groundnuts. It is challenging the elimination of Aflatoxin contamination from the seeds; the entire batch needs to be discarded, resulting in a loss for farmers, which are not being compensated. Aflatoxins contamination is one of the leading causes of economic loss in groundnuts [1]. Maize is a staple food crop widely cultivated in all regions around the globe. Aflatoxin contamination leads to the significant loss of maize kernels. Maize kernels are filled with starch and proteins, a good source for fungal growth, and the plant suffers contamination. Insect activities induce infections.

Contamination can be prevented in the initial stages of infection but must be monitored regularly. Due to aflatoxin-contaminated maize consumption, Kenya had high mortality. A high aflatoxin concentration in food can be lethal and must be impeded by traditional and newly developed technologies [7]. Several technologies have been developed to manage aflatoxins, such as Aflasafe®, Aflaguard®, Hermetic bags, and

PICS bags, which show promising results in reducing contamination [27, 83]. Newer technology, such as Aflascan, was developed by Proscan and ICRISAT researchers. This device can visually detect aflatoxins in groundnuts with a high accuracy level. Coffee consumption is widely spread globally and plays an essential role in the economy with additional health benefits.

Contaminated coffee beans containing aflatoxins can cause aflatoxicosis in humans and animals. There is a need for specific limits on aflatoxin content in food products with accurate monitoring. Many aflatoxin-producing fungi grow in temperate and humid regions during harvest and storage [86]. Aflatoxin contamination causes a massive loss of coffee beans worldwide and affects the economy. Many strategies are used to reduce aflatoxin contents in coffee. However, there are certain limitations to the chemical method, and there is a risk of other diseases due to chemical impurities in coffee. In the traditional method, some aflatoxins are heat-resistant AFB1. Novel techniques need to be developed for the best results. Aflatoxin has a series of global health issues, and it causes hepatic cancer and cirrhosis in humans and animals [6]. Aflatoxin control strategies will provide a better quality of coffee beans and reduce several harmful diseases.

It is a fundamental need to ensure food safety against deadly mycotoxins and aflatoxins. The first limits for aflatoxins were set in the late 1960s. By 2003, many countries had developed their limits for aflatoxins according to their needs. There is a need for research on aflatoxins to explore the short and long-term effects on human health [87].

5. Conclusion

In this review, comprehensive data has been presented from previous studies by researchers. Aflatoxins are a significant issue worldwide; they cause a substantial economic burden on developing countries. It is responsible for contaminating the crops like groundnut, maize, and coffee. These crops are economically important as their never-ending demand in the local and international market makes them perfect crops for trading. *Aspergillus* is soil-borne fungi that produce Aflatoxins in stress conditions caused due to environmental factors. In research of IARC, it was found that aflatoxins have the potential to induce cancer, and they categorize it as a group 1 carcinogen. Groundnut, maize, and coffee are considered commodity crops. They are on the list of 10 highly traded crops, increasing their importance in the market. Due to fungal infections, farmers face huge losses as when aflatoxin is produced in seeds, it cannot be eradicated, and it is very stable, having heat resistance capability. The level of aflatoxin in seeds can be reduced to a certain level by chemical treatments, which are costly and hazardous. Aflatoxins are untraceable and which makes them more dangerous to humans and animals. There are very few solutions available to reduce aflatoxins in crops. Recently, some modified technologies were developed and used in preharvest conditions as a suitable time to stop the infection from fungi like *Aspergillus*. Aflasafe and Aflaguard are genetically developed products that help reduce the aflatoxin-producing *Aspergillus* on farms. Hermetic bags and PICS are technologies utilized in postharvest conditions. These bags are integrated with specific compounds that inhibit fungi infections. Still, even after these technologies are available. Aflatoxins are a concern because this technology can not altogether remove the contamination in seeds; it only prevents them to some extent. Still, further research is needed to find the eco-friendly and less costly methods to eradicate aflatoxins from seeds completely. This study will help develop techniques and technologies to control and manage aflatoxins in preharvest and postharvest conditions.

Acknowledgements

AK acknowledges the support of the UGC NET-JRF Fellowship by University Grant Commissions (UGC), Delhi, India. VBCS greatly acknowledges the support of the CSIR Endophyte Network Project under the FBR Scheme (MLP 0048). The authors acknowledge the support of the Director, CSIR-Central Food Technological Research Institute Mysore (CFTRI), 570020, Karnataka, for providing the necessary facilities. (CSIR-CFTRI Manuscript Communication Number: PMC/2021-22/158).

Author contributions

AK and VBCS conceptualized the topic; AK wrote the manuscript; VBCS & AR corrected the manuscript. The authors read and approved the final manuscript.

Author details

Anup Ramdas Kodape[1,2], Ashika Raveendran[1,2]
and Chikkarasanahalli Shivegowda Vivek Babu[1,2*]

1 Food Protectants and Infestation Control (FPIC) Department, CSIR-Central Food Technological Research Institute (CSIR-CFTRI), Mysuru, Karnataka, India

2 Academy of Scientific and Innovative Research (AcSIR), Ghaziabad, Uttar Pradesh, India

*Address all correspondence to: vivekbabu.cs@cftri.res.in

References

[1] Pickova D, Ostry V, Toman J, Malir F. Aflatoxins: History, significant milestones, recent data on their toxicity and ways to mitigation. Toxins (Basel). 2021;**13**(6):1-23

[2] Kensler TW, Roebuck BD, Wogan GN, Groopman JD. Aflatoxin: A 50-year Odyssey of mechanistic and translational toxicology. Toxicological Sciences. 2011;**120**(Suppl. 1):28-48

[3] Imdad A, Mullany LC, Baqui AH, et al. The effect of umbilical cord cleansing with chlorhexidine on omphalitis and neonatal mortality in community settings in developing countries: A meta-analysis. BMC Public Health. 2013;13:S15. DOI: 10.1186/1471-2458-13-S3-S15

[4] Mallick L, Yourkavitch J, Allen C. Trends, determinants, and newborn mortality related to thermal care and umbilical cord care practices in South Asia. BMC Pediatrics. 2019;19:248. DOI: 10.1186/s12887-019-1616-2

[5] Nesbitt BF, O'kelly J, Sargeant K, Ann S. Aspergillus flavus and turkey X disease: Toxic metabolites of aspergillus flavus. Nature. 1962;**195**(4846): 1062-1063. DOI: 10.1038/1951062a0

[6] Liu Y, Wu F. Global burden of Aflatoxin-induced hepatocellular carcinoma: A risk assessment. Environmental Health Perspectives. 2010;**118**(6):818-824

[7] Los A, Ziuzina D, Boehm D, Cullen PJ, Bourkea P, Agriopoulou S, et al. Control strategies: Prevention and detoxification in foods. Food. 2020;**86**(9):137

[8] Sahil VP, Tejas CB, Hiren NB, Pratibha S, Abhay K. Aflatoxins: Causes & effects. Agrobios Newsletter. 2015;13:140-142

[9] Available from: https://www.fssai.gov.in/upload/advisories/2020/12/5fca3db8df192Order_Revised_Manual_Mycotoxins_04_12_2020.pdf

[10] Kumar D, Kalita P. Reducing postharvest losses during storage of grain crops to strengthen food security in developing countries. Food. 2017;**6**(1):1-22

[11] Shukla GN, Kumar A, Jha A, Singh N, Sharma P, Singh J, et al. Maize Vision. Fed Indian Chambers Commer Ind. 2022;**2019**:1-92

[12] Cotty PJ, Mellon JE. Ecology of aflatoxin producing fungi and biocontrol of aflatoxin contamination. Mycotoxin Research. 2006;**22**(2):110-117

[13] Ngindu A, Kenya PR, Ocheng DM, Omondi TN, Ngare W, Gatei D, et al. Outbreak of acute hepatitis caused by aflatoxin poisoning in kenya. Lancet. 1982;**319**(8285):1346-1348

[14] Grimaud P, Sserunjogi ML, Grillet N. Ajfand. 2007;7(5):1-15. DOI: 10.18697/ajfand.16.2750

[15] Gnonlonfin GJB, Hell K, Adjovi Y, Fandohan P, Koudande DO, Mensah GA, et al. A review on aflatoxin contamination and its implications in the developing world: A sub-saharan african perspective. Critical Reviews in Food Science and Nutrition. 2013;**53**(4):349-365

[16] Care T, Malhotra P, Malhotra V, Ps G, Gupta U, Sanwariya Y. Epidemiological profile and clinical spectrum of hepatitis B-Ten years japanese journal of gastroenterology and hepatology epidemiological profile and clinical spectrum of hepatitis B-ten years

experience at tertiary care centre of northeren India. 2021

[17] Wogan GN, Paglialunga S, Newberne PM. Carcinogenic effects of low dietary levels of aflatoxin B1 in rats. Food and Cosmetics Toxicology. Oct 1974;12(5-6):681-685. DOI: 10.1016/0015-6264(74)90239-9

[18] IARC. AFLATOXINS (IARC Summary and Evaluation, Volume 82, 2002) [Internet]. 2002. Available from: http://www.inchem.org/documents/iarc/vol82/82-04.html

[19] Norlia M, Jinap S, Nor-Khaizura MAR, Radu S, Samsudin NIP, Azri FA. Aspergillus section flavi and aflatoxins: Occurrence, detection, and identification in raw peanuts and peanut-based products along the supply chain. Frontiers in Microbiology. 2019;**10**(November):1-17

[20] Stern MC, Umbach DM, Yu MC, London SJ, Zhang Z, Taylor JA. Hepatitis B, Aflatoxin B 1, and p53 Codon 249 mutation in hepatocellular carcinomas from Guangxi, People' s Republic of China, and a Meta-analysis of Existing Studies 1. 2001;**10**(June):617-625

[21] Denissenko MF, Koudriakova TB, Smith L, O'Connor TR, Riggs AD, Pfeifer GP. The p53 codon 249 Mutational Hotspot in Hepatocellular Carcinoma is not Related to Selective Formation or Persistence of aflatoxin B 1 Adducts. 10 Dec 1998;17(23):3007-3014. DOI: 10.1038/sj.onc.1202214. PMID: 9881702

[22] Hesseltine CW, Shotwell OL, Ellis JJ, Stubblefield RD. Aflatoxin formation by Aspergillus flavus. Bacteriological Reviews. 1966;**30**(4):795-805

[23] Yabe MK. Enzyme Reactions and Genes in Aflatoxin Biosynthesis. Applied Microbiology and Biotechnology. 2004;64(6):745-755. DOI: 10.1007/s00253-004-1566-x. Epub 2004 Mar 12. PMID: 15022028.

[24] Jallow A, Xie H, Tang X, Qi Z, Li P. Worldwide aflatoxin contamination of agricultural products and foods: From occurrence to control. Comprehensive Reviews in Food Science and Food Safety. 2021;**20**(3):2332-2381

[25] Soni P, Gangurde SS, Ortega-Beltran A, Kumar R, Parmar S, Sudini HK, et al. Functional biology and molecular mechanisms of host-pathogen interactions for aflatoxin contamination in groundnut (Arachis hypogaea L.) and maize (Zea mays L.). Frontiers in Microbiology. 2020;**11**(March):1-22

[26] Practices PM, Pandey MK, Kumar R, Pandey AK, Soni P, Gangurde SS, et al. Mitigating aflatoxin contamination in groundnut through a combination of genetic resistance and post-harvest management practices. Toxins (Basel). 3 Jun 2019;11(6):315. DOI: 10.3390/toxins11060315. PMID: 31163657; PMCID: PMC6628460

[27] Bandyopadhyay R, Ortega-Beltran A, Akande A, Mutegi C, Atehnkeng J, Kaptoge L, et al. Biological control of aflatoxins in Africa: Current status and potential challenges in the face of climate change. World Mycotoxin Journal. 2016;**9**(5):771-789

[28] Tariq Alam SR. Management of aflatoxins in peanut. 2020;**1**:1-9

[29] Available from: https://www.researchgate.net/publication/262451496_Groundnut_aflatoxin_and_its_management

[30] Shad MA, Perveez H, Nawaz H, Khan H, Ullah MA. Evaluation of biochemical and phytochemical composition of some groundnut varieties

grown in arid zone of Pakistan. Pakistan Journal of Botany. 2009;**41**(6):2739-2749

[31] Panche AN, Diwan AD, Chandra SR. Flavonoids: An overview. Journal of Nutritional Science. 29 Dec 2016;5:e47. DOI: 10.1017/jns.2016.41. PMID: 28620474; PMCID: PMC5465813

[32] Awad AB, Chan KC, Downie AC, Fink CS. Peanuts as a source of beta-sitosterol, a sterol with anticancer properties. Nutrition and Cancer. 2000;**36**(2):238-241

[33] Bhatnagar D, Cary JW, Ehrlich K, Yu J, Cleveland TE. Understanding the genetics of regulation of aflatoxin production and Aspergillus flavus development. Mycopathologia. 2006;**162**(3):155-166

[34] Eskola M, Kos G, Elliott CT, Hajšlová J, Mayar S, Krska R. Worldwide contamination of food-crops with mycotoxins: Validity of the widely cited 'FAO estimate' of 25%. Critical Reviews in Food Science and Nutrition. 2020;**60**(16):2773-2789

[35] Agbetiameh D, Ortega-Beltran A, Awuah RT, Atehnkeng J, Cotty PJ, Bandyopadhyay R. Prevalence of aflatoxin contamination in maize and groundnut in Ghana: Population structure, distribution, and toxigenicity of the causal agents. Plant Disease. 2018;**102**(4):764-772

[36] Omotayo OP, Omotayo AO, Mwanza M, Babalola OO. Prevalence of mycotoxins and their consequences on human health. Toxicology Research. 2019;**35**(1):1-7

[37] Mitchell NJ, Bowers E, Hurburgh C, Wu F. Potential economic losses to the US corn industry from aflatoxin contamination. Food Addit Contam—Part A. Chem Anal Control Expo Risk Assess. 2016;**33**(3):540-550. DOI: 10.1080/19440049.2016.1138545

[38] Rewards M. A Conceptual Framework for Conducting Country and Economic Assessment of Aflatoxin Contamination. Volume I. Contract # Add the extension. I:1-20

[39] Nyandieka HS, Maina JO, Nyamwange C. Destruction of aflatoxins in contaminated maize samples using ammoniation procedures. East and Central African Journal of Pharmaceutical Sciences. 2009;12(3)

[40] Whitlow L. Evaluation of mycotoxin binders. In: Proc 4th Mid-Atlantic Nutr .... 2006. pp. 132-143. Available from: http://manc.umd.edu/documents/2006_complete_proceedings.pdf#page=138

[41] Mamo FT, Abate BA, Tesfaye K, Nie C, Wang G, Liu Y. Mycotoxins in ethiopia: A review on prevalence, economic and health impacts. Toxins (Basel). 2020;**12**(10):1-21

[42] Duangpapeng P, Ketthaisong D, Lomthaisong K, Lertrat K, Scott MP, Suriharn B. Corn Tassel: A new source of phytochemicals and antioxidant potential for value-added product development in the agro-industry. Agronomy. 2018;**8**(11):242. DOI: 10.3390/agronomy8110242

[43] Gökcen BB, Şanlier N. Coffee consumption and disease correlations. Critical Reviews in Food Science and Nutrition. 2019;59(2):336-348

[44] Marcucci C, Dias R, Almeida M, Benassi M. Antioxidant activity of commercial soluble coffees. Beverages. 2017;**3**(4):27

[45] Bajaj D, Ballal S. A Review on Antioxidant Activity of Coffee and Its Additives. 2021;**33**:77-85

[46] George SE, Ramalakshmi K, Rao LJM. A perception on health

benefits of coffee. Critical Reviews in Food Science and Nutrition. 2008;**48**(5):464-486

[47] Cornelis MC. The impact of caffeine and coffee on human health. Nutrients. 2019;**11**(2):11-14

[48] Zakir Z, Hassan M. Caffeine (1, 3, 7-Trimethylxanthine): The good and the bad: A Review and the Bad: A review. International Journal of Health and Biological Sciences. 2013;**2**(4):313-323

[49] Heckman MA, Weil J, de Mejia EG. Caffeine (1, 3, 7-trimethylxanthine) in foods: A comprehensive review on consumption, functionality, safety, and regulatory matters. Journal of Food Science. 2010;**75**(3):R77-R87. DOI: 10.1111/j.1750-3841.2010.01561.x. PMID: 20492310

[50] Turner PC. The molecular epidemiology of chronic aflatoxin driven impaired child growth. Scientifica (Cairo). 2016;**2013**(2013):1-21

[51] Planning Committee for a Workshop on Potential Health Hazards Associated with Consumption of Caffeine in Food and Dietary Supplements; Food and Nutrition Board; Board on Health Sciences Policy; Institute of Medicine. Caffeine in Food and Dietary Supplements: Examining Safety: Workshop Summary. Washington (DC): National Academies Press (US); 23 Apr 2014. Available from: https://www.ncbi.nlm.nih.gov/books/NBK202230/ DOI: 10.17226/18607

[52] Higdon JV, Frei B. Coffee and health: A review of recent human research. Critical Reviews in Food Science and Nutrition. 2006;**46**(2):101-123

[53] Arnesen E, Huseby NE, Brenn T, Try K. The Tromsø heart study: Distribution of, and determinants for, gamma-glutamyltransferase in a free-living population. Scandinavian Journal of Clinical and Laboratory Investigation. 1986 Feb;**46**(1):63-70

[54] Heath RD, Brahmbhatt M, Tahan AC, Ibdah JA, Tahan V. Coffee: The magical bean for liver diseases. World Journal of Hepatology. 2017;**9**(15):689-696

[55] Liu F, Wang X, Wu G, Chen L, Hu P, Ren H. Coffee Consumption Decreases Risks for Hepatic Fibrosis and Cirrhosis: A Meta-Analysis. 2015;**73**:1-13

[56] Kumar V, Kaur J, Panghal A, Kaur S, Handa V. Caffeine: A boon or bane. Nutrition & Food Science. 2018;**48**(1):61-75

[57] Messina G, Zannella C, Monda V, Dato A, Liccardo D, De Blasio S, et al. The beneficial effects of coffee in human nutrition. Biologie et Médecine. 2015;**7**:1-5

[58] Kim Y, Jhon YK, D-Y. Changes of the chlorogenic acid, caffeine, gama-aminobutyric acid (GABA) and antioxdant activities during germination of coffee bean (Coffea arabica). Emirates Journal of Food and Agriculture. 2018;**30**(8):675

[59] Jeon JS, Kim HT, Jeong IH, Hong SR, Oh MS, Yoon MH, et al. Contents of chlorogenic acids and caffeine in various coffee-related products. Journal of Advanced Research. 2019;**17**:85-94. DOI: 10.1016/j.jare.2019.01.002

[60] Tajik N, Tajik M, Mack I, Enck P. The potential effects of chlorogenic acid, the main phenolic components in coffee, on health: A comprehensive review of the literature. European Journal of Nutrition. 2017;**56**(7):2215-2244

[61] Cavin C, Holzhaeuser D, Scharf G, Constable A, Huber WW, Schilter B.

Cafestol and kahweol, two coffee specific diterpenes with anti-carcinogenic activity. Food and Chemical Toxicology. 2002;**40**(8):1155-1163

[62] Pereira LFP, Ivamoto ST. Chapter 6 - characterization of coffee genes involved in isoprenoid and diterpene metabolic pathways. In: Preedy VR, editor. Coffee in Health and Disease Prevention. Academic Press; 2015. pp. 45-51. DOI: 10.1016/B978-0-12-409517-5.00006-1. ISBN 9780124095175

[63] Post SM, De Wit ECM, Princen HMG. Cafestol, the cholesterol-raising factor in boiled coffee, suppresses bile acid synthesis by downregulation of cholesterol 7α-hydroxylase and sterol 27-hydroxylase in rat hepatocytes. Arteriosclerosis, Thrombosis, and Vascular Biology. 1997;**17**(11):3064-3070

[64] Wasim S, Kukkar V, Awad VM, Sakhamuru S, Malik BH. Neuroprotective and neurodegenerative aspects of coffee and its active ingredients in view of scientific literature. Cureus. 5 Aug 2020;12(8):e9578. DOI: 10.7759/cureus.9578. PMID: 32923185; PMCID: PMC7478584

[65] Saeed M, Naveed M, BiBi J, Ali Kamboh A, Phil L, Chao S. Potential nutraceutical and food additive properties and risks of coffee: A comprehensive overview. Critical Reviews in Food Science and Nutrition. 2019;**59**(20):3293-3319. DOI: 10.1080/10408398.2018.1489368

[66] Velazquez Pereda Mdel C, Dieamant Gde C, Eberlin S, Nogueira C, Colombi D, Di Stasi LC, et al. Effect of green Coffea arabica L. seed oil on extracellular matrix components and water-channel expression in in vitro and ex vivo human skin models. Journal of Cosmetic Dermatology. 2009;**8**(1):56-62. DOI: 10.1111/j.1473-2165.2009.00425.x

[67] Del M, Velazquez C, Dieamant GDC, Eberlin S, Nogueira C, Colombi D, et al. Effect of green Coffea arabica L. seed oil on extracellular matrix components and water-channel expression in in vitro and ex vivo human skin models. 2009;56-62

[68] Birch AJ. Biosynthesis of polyketides and related compounds. Science. 1967;**156**(3772):202-206

[69] Liao J, He Z, Xia Y, Lei Y, Liao B. A review on biosynthesis and genetic regulation of aflatoxin production by major Aspergillus fungi. Oil Crop Science. 2020;**5**(4):166-173. DOI: 10.1016/j.ocsci.2020.11.001

[70] Khan R, Ghazali FM, Mahyudin NA, Samsudin NIP. Aflatoxin biosynthesis, genetic regulation, toxicity, and control strategies: A review. Journal of Fungi 2021;7:606. DOI: 10.3390/jof7080606

[71] Watanabe CMH, Townsend CA. Initial characterization of a type I fatty acid synthase and polyketide synthase multienzyme complex NorS in the biosynthesis of aflatoxin B(1). Chemistry & Biology. 2002 Sep;**9**(9):981-988

[72] Moon YS, Kim L, Chun HS, Lee SE. 4-hydroxy-7-methyl-3-phenylcoumarin suppresses aflatoxin biosynthesis via downregulation of aflk expressing versicolorin B synthase in aspergillus flavus. Molecules. 29 Apr 2017;**22**(5):712. DOI: 10.3390/molecules22050712. PMID: 28468270; PMCID: PMC6154296

[73] Yabe K, Nakajima H. Enzyme reactions and genes in aflatoxin biosynthesis. Applied Microbiology and Biotechnology. Jun 2004;**64**(6):745-755. DOI: 10.1007/s00253-004-1566-x. Epub 2004 Mar 12. PMID: 15022028

[74] Sakuno E, Wen Y, Hatabayashi H, Arai H, Aoki C, Yabe K, et al. Aspergillus parasiticus cyclase catalyzes two

dehydration steps in aflatoxin biosynthesis. Applied and Environmental Microbiology. 2005;**71**(6):2999-3006

[75] Singh BP, Rateb ME, Rodriguez-Couto S, Polizeli MdLTdM, Li W-J. Editorial: Microbial secondary metabolites: Recent developments and technological challenges. Frontiers in Microbiology. 2019;10:914. DOI: 10.3389/fmicb.2019.00914

[76] Liang N, Kitts DD. Antioxidant property of coffee components: Assessment of methods that define mechanisms of action. 19 Nov 2014;19(11):19180-19208. DOI: 10.3390/molecules191119180. PMID: 25415479; PMCID: PMC6270823

[77] Yu J. Current understanding on aflatoxin biosynthesis and future perspective in reducing aflatoxin contamination. Toxins (Basel). 2012;**4**(11):1024-1057

[78] Ehrlich KC, Chang PK, Scharfenstein LL, Cary JW, Crawford JM, Townsend CA. Absence of the aflatoxin biosynthesis gene, norA, allows accumulation of deoxyaflatoxin B1 in Aspergillus flavus cultures. FEMS Microbiology Letters. 2010;**305**(1):65-70

[79] Senghor LA, Ortega-Beltran A, Atehnkeng J, Callicott KA, Cotty PJ, BandyopadhyayR.Theatoxigenicbiocontrol product Aflasafe SN01 is a valuable tool to mitigate aflatoxin contamination of both maize and groundnut cultivated in Senegal. Plant Disease. 2020;**104**(2):510-520

[80] Raveau R, Fontaine J, Lounès-Hadj SA. Essential oils as potential alternative biocontrol products against plant pathogens and weeds: A review. Food. 21 Mar 2020;**9**(3):365. DOI: 10.3390/foods9030365. PMID: 32245234; PMCID: PMC7143296

[81] Available from: https://assets.greenbook.net/M92685.pdf

[82] Indoors U. Keep out of reach of children. Environmental Hazards. 2015;**8536**:3-4

[83] Baributsa D, Njoroge AW. The use and profitability of hermetic technologies for grain storage among smallholder farmers in eastern Kenya. Journal of Stored Products Research. 2020;**87**:101618. DOI: 10.1016/j.jspr.2020.101618

[84] Murdock LL, Baoua IB. On purdue improved cowpea storage (PICS) technology: Background, mode of action, future prospects. Journal of Stored Products Research. 2014;**58**:3-11. DOI: 10.1016/j.jspr.2014.02.006

[85] Available from: https://purescanai.com/

[86] Kumar P, Mahato DK, Kamle M, Mohanta TK, Kang SG. Aflatoxins: A global concern for food safety, human health and their management. Frontiers in Microbiology. 2017;**7**(Jan):1-10

[87] Lire WH. Review on health benefit and risk of coffee consumption. Medicinal and Aromatic Plants Research Journals. 2017;**06**. DOI: 10.4172/2155-9821.1000301

Chapter 5

Aflatoxin and Mycotoxin Analysis: An Overview Including Options for Resource-limited Settings

Godfrey Z. Magoke, Robyn G. Alders, Mark Krockenberger and Wayne L. Bryden

Abstract

Aflatoxins are fungal toxins of serious human health concern, more so in some developing countries where significant contamination of staple foods occurs and the prevalence of aflatoxin-related health effects is high. A plethora of techniques for food mycotoxin testing has been developed. Modern chromatographic techniques allow quantitative determination with high accuracy and sensitivity, but are expensive and difficult to operate and maintain. Rapid tests provide a cheaper alternative for screening large numbers of samples, although they need validation on all food matrices that are tested. One important aspect of tackling aflatoxin contamination and exposure is to ensure the availability of suitable methods for detection and quantification that are rapid, sensitive, accurate, robust, and cost-effective for food surveillance in resource-limited settings.

Keywords: mycotoxins, analysis, food safety, rapid tests

1. Introduction

Food contamination with mycotoxins is a serious human health concern worldwide and of greatest significance in developing countries [1, 2]. Of all the mycotoxins, aflatoxins are more toxic, widespread in nature, and have been associated with significant health effects in humans and reduced productivity in farmed animals [3–5]. Recent estimates suggest that 60–80% of crops contain detectable concentrations of mycotoxins. In many instances, there is co-contamination with more than one toxin and this is geographically dependent on climate and farming practices [6, 7].

Aflatoxins affect approximately 4.5 billion people in developing countries, causing acute fatal hepatitis in individuals exposed to highly contaminated grains. Low level, chronic exposure to aflatoxins is associated with the development of liver cancer in adults, reduced immunity, and lowered growth and stunting in infants and children [8–10]. Monitoring food for contamination with aflatoxins is essential, although a number of challenges must be faced, including low concentrations and variable distribution of the toxin in contaminated grains within storage facilities. These factors will contribute to variable test results as well as issues related to test sensitivity and specificity in varied food matrices [5, 11].

This chapter provides an overview of sample extraction and cleanup procedures, together with analytical techniques developed for mycotoxins, including aflatoxins. The advantages and disadvantages of the different approaches affecting suitability for use in aflatoxin food surveillance and quantitative confirmation are outlined. In developing countries, rapid tests make a significant contribution to aflatoxin control and a perspective on their application in resource-limited settings is given.

2. General mycotoxin analytical techniques

Mycotoxins present a great analytical challenge. Not only do they include a diversity of chemical compounds, but are heterogeneously distributed at varying concentrations in a wide range of agricultural commodities, foods, feeds, and biological samples that require specific extraction, cleanup, separation, and detection methods [11]. Some mycotoxins, especially deoxynivalenol and zearalenone, are conjugated as a result of plant metabolism, and these "masked" mycotoxins may contribute 20% of total of the parent mycotoxin but are not detected during conventional analysis [5, 11].

Quantification of mycotoxins requires expensive laboratory equipment that needs well-trained personnel to operate [12], as well as involving a series of steps and procedures that may be laborious and time-consuming [11]. The need for high sensitivity tests to detect the minimum levels of the mycotoxin possible for regulatory purposes, coupled with rapidity, high accuracy, simplicity, robustness, and selectivity have been the main driving forces behind the improvement and development of new mycotoxin analytical protocols [11, 13]. Mycotoxin analysis is essential to quantify the toxin for risk evaluation, diagnosis, and monitoring mitigation strategies [5].

3. Sampling

Sampling for aflatoxin determination in food commodities poses a particular challenge given uneven toxin distribution and the low levels at which mycotoxins occur [5]. As a result, some national and international food safety authorities and organizations have prescribed sampling methods for various food commodities for the purpose of achieving representative samples that may be used to determine concentrations of various mycotoxins in foodstuffs for official control purposes; sampling is potentially the biggest source of error in mycotoxin testing [14]. For many commodities, detailed sampling plans have been devised [15]. To obtain a representative sample from a grain storage facility, for example, incremental samples have to be taken from different places of the facility [11] with the entire primary sample ground, mixed, and subsampled to ensure that the analyzed portion has a similar toxin concentration as the original sample [11, 16].

4. Analytical procedures

Analytical procedures for mycotoxins entail extraction from the matrix with a suitable solvent, cleanup of co-extracted matrix components, and identification/

quantification of the toxin using suitable analytical facilities [12, 17]. Some exceptional techniques, such as infra-red spectroscopy, may detect mycotoxin contamination directly in ground samples without prior solvent extraction or cleanup but are limited to screening purposes because of high matrix interference and lack of suitable calibration materials [11]. Although additional cleanup is essential for chromatographic determination, the diluted extracts may be directly used with immunoanalytical methods [13].

5. Sample extraction

Extraction liberates the mycotoxin from the sample matrix with subsequent extract cleanup to reduce matrix interference, hence improving the sensitivity and robustness of the technique [11, 18]. Depending on the physicochemical properties of the mycotoxins and sample matrix, various combinations of extraction solvents may be used [11]. Relatively polar solvents, such as methanol, acetone, acetonitrile, ethyl acetate, diethyl ether, 1-octanol, toluene, dichloromethane, chloroform, or a mixture of them, may provide efficient extraction of mycotoxins, with minimal addition of water and acid solution helping to enhance extraction efficiency [19, 20]. A suitable extraction solvent should only remove the mycotoxins from the sample with high efficiency as well as being cheap, safe to use, and reduce matrix interference. For this purpose, mixtures of methanol-water and acetonitrile-water at appropriate ratios are the most frequently used extraction solvents for mycotoxin analysis [20].

Other parameters, such as sample/extractive solvent ratio, temperature, and time of extraction, may affect the extraction process; therefore, need to be carefully controlled to achieve accurate quantification [16]. High temperature and pressure instruments, such as accelerated solvent extraction/pressurized liquid extraction and microwave-assisted extraction methods hasten the process by speeding up and automating the extraction, use less solvent and provide better extraction efficiencies (in terms of extraction yield and/or recovery) compared to classical solvent extraction techniques. However, they are limited by the high cost of the equipment and may not be suitable for thermally unstable analytes [11, 16]. Non-polar solvents, such as hexane and cyclohexane, may be used before or following the extraction procedure to remove lipids in certain sample types, for example, groundnuts and maize [16, 19]. The presence of pigments, essential oils, and fatty acids in some samples may make extraction difficult and necessitate the use of different extraction solvents, such as a mixture of ethyl acetate-formic acid [20]. Chlorinated solvents are considered to be toxic and ecologically harmful, hence should be avoided, where possible in the extraction process [12]. Deep eutectic solvent has been recently reported as an environmentally safe extraction solvent limiting the use of traditional solvents and derivatization reagents [20].

Extraction is usually enabled by the high-speed blending of ground sample-extraction solvent mixture or employing a mechanical shaker followed by filtration before subsequent purification step, where applicable [19]. Evaluation of extraction procedures based on methanol-water and acetone-water in maize found [21] that the acetone-water mixture (6 + 4 v/v) showed the best extraction efficiency for all aflatoxins (B_1, B_2, G_1, and G_2) compared to the commonly used mixtures of methanol-water (8 + 2 v/v) or acetone-water (85 + 15 v/v).

Purification of sample extracts is required to reduce matrix-induced signal suppression or enhancement in mycotoxin detection [11, 19, 22]. Immunoaffinity columns (IAC), solid-phase extraction (SPE), column chromatography, multi-functional columns, and liquid-liquid partitioning (LLE) may be used for purification purposes with the purified sample reconstituted in a suitable solvent before chromatographic analysis [13].

5.1 Solvent extraction methods

5.1.1 Liquid extraction/partitioning

Liquid extraction or partitioning is a common and arguably the simplest method of sample purification relying on the solubility of the target compounds in a particular solvent, and the insolubility of competing or interfering compounds in the same solvent [18].

5.1.2 Liquid-liquid partitioning/extraction

Liquid-liquid extraction (LLE) is used repetitively to extract analytes quantitatively by concentrating those analytes that migrate between two partitioned immiscible solvents [19]. In LLE, traditional solvents with a low dielectric constant (those that tend to be immiscible with water) are poor at extracting polar compounds, including most mycotoxins. Suitable solvents, such as methanol or acetonitrile, should be mixed with water in the presence of salts to reduce the mutual miscibility, allowing the polar analytes to move selectively into the polar organic phase from the aqueous phase [18]. Solvents, such as hexane and cyclohexane, for example, may be used to remove non-polar contaminants, for example, lipids and cholesterol through liquid-liquid extraction [23]. However, the method is used infrequently because it is labor intensive, uses vast amounts of solvent, leads to losses, and is time-consuming [13, 19].

5.1.3 Dispersive liquid-liquid microextraction

Dispersive liquid-liquid microextraction (DLLME) is a recently introduced miniaturized extraction procedure. The technique is based on the formation of a cloudy solution consisting of fine droplets of the extractant solvent dispersed entirely in the aqueous (continuous) phase. This occurs following the rapid addition of a mixture of a water-immiscible extractant solvent, and a water-miscible dispersive solvent into an aqueous solution containing the analytes. As a result of a very large surface area formed by the dispersed extractant micro-droplets, the analytes are rapidly and efficiently enriched in the extractive solvent and, after centrifugation, can be separated in the sediment phase [16, 24].

This technique is cheap, environmentally safe, simple, fast, and efficient [16]. However, it is difficult to automate and necessitates using a third component (disperser solvent), which commonly decreases the partition coefficient of analytes into the extractant solvent [24].

5.1.4 Vortex-assisted liquid-liquid microextraction

Vortex-assisted liquid-liquid microextraction is a new equilibrium-based solvent microextraction technique. It is based on the dispersion of micro-droplets of the extraction solvent into the aqueous sample and is achieved by vortex agitation, forming a mild emulsification process [24, 25]. Separation of the two phases occurs upon centrifugation, with the floating extractant phase restoring its original single micro drop shape; it is easily collected with the help of a microsyringe and used for HPLC analysis [24, 26].

Several experimental parameters, namely, organic solvent, agitation time, rotational speed of the vortex agitator, acceptor phase volume, aqueous sample volume, pH, and salt addition may affect the extraction process, and these need to be controlled and optimized for optimum performance of the procedure [24]. Surfactants, such as Triton X-114, Tween-20, Triton X-100, and cetyltrimethylammonium bromide (CTAB), may be used to enhance extraction efficiency [25].

This technique is rapid, as the fine droplets formed, extract target analytes toward equilibrium faster because of the shorter diffusion distance and larger specific surface area compared to the DLLME where the need for a disperser solvent is mandatory [24, 26].

5.1.5 Dilute and shoot method

The dilute-and-shoot (DaS) method utilizes the improved sensitivity and robustness of modern equipment. It is based on dilution followed by direct injection of samples that are presumed to be inherently clean enough to not require full preparation, thus reducing cost. It has the benefits of rapidity, can work with multiple analytes, and limits the potential loss of analyte due to pretreatment, although it still has a risk of matrix interference that can overwhelm instrument sensitivity [18].

5.2 Solid-phase extraction methods

5.2.1 Solid-phase extraction

The solid-phase extraction (SPE) technique utilizes small disposable cartridges packed with silica gel or bonded phases that are in the stationary phase to bind impurities or target analytes. The impurities can be washed off, and the analyte recovered using a suitable rinse solution [19, 23, 27].

In SPE, the aqueous sample extract is applied to the conditioned column followed by rinsing to remove matrix compounds, with the analyte eluted from the column using an organic solvent. Evaporation of excessive solvent can be employed for further concentration [13, 19].

Compared to LLE, SPE has the advantage of rapidity, efficiency, reproducibility, uses considerably less solvent, and offers a wide range of selectivity, however, it is limited by the fact that there is no single fit-for-all cartridge [19, 23].

5.2.2 Ion-exchange columns

Ion-exchange columns use ionic materials, such as SAX (strong anion exchange) in SPE to extract mycotoxins that present as ions, such as moniliformin, in aqueous solutions. The target molecule is bound to charged groups on the silica material and removed by the addition of a strong ionic solution because of its higher affinity to the sorbent or by the altered pH [19, 23].

5.2.3 Matrix solid-phase dispersion

Matrix solid-phase dispersion (MSPD) utilizes some SPE sorbent materials (usually octadecyl silica, silica gel, or alumina) that is ground typically with 1 g of a homogenized sample using a pestle and mortar. The solid mixture is then transferred to a glass column or cartridge containing a lower layer of co-sorbent material, such as carbon black, with the adsorbed residues selectively eluted with an appropriate solvent [16, 28, 29]. This technique has the advantages of flexibility and versatility and can be used in a single step with small amounts of sorbent and solvent, thus reducing the cost and time of analysis. However, it is not easily automated, often requiring an additional cleanup step that could be time-consuming for a large number of samples [16, 29].

5.2.4 Solid-phase microextraction

Solid-phase microextraction (SPME) combines extraction and concentration of analytes in a single step and is based on the extraction of analytes by adsorption to a thin fiber coated with different stationary phases. This is followed by thermal desorption into a heated injector for gas chromatography or with a solvent when liquid chromatography is used [16]. It is simple, safe, and has a wide application on polar and non-polar compounds [30]. However, it has the disadvantage of high cost, fiber fragility, and is susceptible to experimental conditions that can affect reproducibility and sensitivity [16, 31].

5.2.5 Micro-solid phase extraction

The recently introduced micro-solid phase extraction (μ-SPE) uses a sorbent material trapped in a porous membrane sheet to extract the analyte diffusing through it, the μ-SPE device tumbling to stir the process facilitating the mass transfer. Following extraction, desorption is carried out by ultrasonification with the extraction device immersed in a suitable organic solvent. The technique is simple as extraction and cleanup steps are carried out simultaneously and it uses less solvent and sorbent materials [30].

5.2.6 Magnetic solid-phase extraction

Magnetic solid-phase extraction (MSPE) is a new SPE technique that is based on the use of magnetic nanoparticles that are dispersed into the sample solution with separation effected by applying an external magnetic field outside the sample solution [31]. The technique avoids time-consuming column or filtration operations encountered in SPE with the large contact area between the adsorbent and the analyte ensuring a fast mass transfer, which guarantees high extraction efficiency compared to the SPME technique [31, 32].

5.2.7 Immunoaffinity columns

Immunoaffinity columns (IACs) are increasingly used for the cleanup and enrichment of sample extracts [11]. The column containing mycotoxin-specific antibodies bound to solid phase support within the cartridge selectively binds the mycotoxin in the extract. Mycotoxin desorption is achieved using a miscible solvent or by antibody denaturation [16, 19].

Compared to traditional solid-phase cleanup techniques, IAC is more sensitive, specific, easy to use, rapid, safe (minimizes use of hazardous solvents), and robust in terms of applicability to different matrices. However, columns are single-use, more expensive, suffer from storage limitations and stability problems regarding organic solvents, and the possibility of nonspecific interactions due to cross-reactivity with other mycotoxins [11, 12, 16, 19]. However, there is now a commercially available immunoaffinity column ('Myco 6in1'; Vicam, Milford, MA, USA) that may be used in a cleanup procedure for simultaneous determination of multiple mycotoxins [33] that helps mitigate the single use of these IACs.

5.2.8 MycoSep®/Multisep® columns

Mycosep® /Multisep® columns contain selected adsorbents packed in a plastic tube to recover individual mycotoxins from a sample extract [23]. Despite the practicability of the method, the columns are designed per analyte, hence not suitable for multi-toxin determination and may not provide effective purification for some matrixes [16, 23].

5.2.9 Molecular imprinted polymers and aptamers

Synthetic systems, such as molecular imprinted polymers (MIPs), aptamers, and peptides, have been developed to counter shortcomings related to the use of antibodies in IACs [20].

The molecular Imprinted Polymer (MIP) is a synthetic material providing an artificially generated three-dimensional network that is able to specifically rebind a target molecule. It is a cheaper alternative for mycotoxin cleanup and preconcentration as well as affording chemical and thermal stability and solvent compatibility, which is contrary to immunoaffinity columns [11, 34].

During molecular imprinting, cross-linked polymers are formed by free-radical co-polymerization of functional monomers. The cross-linking occurs in the presence of an analyte serving as a template followed by template removal by liquid extraction (washing). This leaves highly selective three-dimensional binding pockets complementary in size, shape, and functionality to the imprinted molecule remaining in the polymer matrix [13]. Despite offering promise for future application, MIP may still be affected by the low specificity and robustness of the technique in terms of kinetics, reuse, ability to withstand unfavorable solvents, and potential sample contamination by template bleeding [23].

On the other hand, aptamers are small fragments of oligonucleotide sequences (single-stranded DNA or RNA), usually containing 10 to 100 bases that bind to their targets by folding into specific three-dimensional structures [35]. Compared to antibodies, they are cheap, stable, reversible, not limited by immunogenicity of targets, and do not require immunization of animals during production [35]. Although difficult to develop, they provide an important avenue for exploitation in mycotoxin cleanup procedures and in sensing instruments [20, 35].

5.2.10 QuEChERS extraction/cleanup

QuEChERS (quick, easy, cheap, effective, rugged, and safe) as a sample pretreatment technique entails solvent extraction, partitioning with magnesium sulfate and other salts, such as NaCl, and cleanup using a dispersive solid-phase extraction (d-SPE) sorbent, especially the primary secondary amine (PSA) and extract centrifugation before analysis [36]. Magnesium sulfate along with NaCl is used to reduce water in the sample during extraction, while PSA retains co-extracted compounds during cleaning [16]. This procedure is simple, rapid, cost-effective, and enables multi-residue determination [16, 36]. The use of QuEChERS is becoming a popular alternative to the dilute-and-shoot approach for multi-mycotoxin determination using LC/MS-based techniques to reduce matrix interference [37]. However, it should be noted that the several QuEChERS commercial kits or QuEChERS-like protocols differ in extraction, partitioning, or dispersive solid-phase extraction (dSPE) steps. They, therefore, may show different cleanup efficiencies, and for optimization an additional cleanup step may be needed to improve the performance of QuEChERS protocols [38].

6. Toxin determination

6.1 Conventional analytical techniques

Conventional analytical methods employ chromatographic separation, particularly, liquid chromatography (LC), thin layer chromatography (TLC) and gas chromatography (GC) coupled to a detection system, with high-performance liquid chromatography (HPLC) after immunoaffinity cleanup combined with fluorescence detection (FLD) or mass spectrometry (MS) frequently employed for the quantitative determination of regulated mycotoxins in food [11, 18].

6.1.1 Thin layer chromatography

Thin layer chromatography (TLC) was traditionally the most widely used mycotoxin screening technique that did not require expensive equipment and enabled high sample throughput [23]. The TLC techniques lack separating power that limits discrimination of co-extracted interference from the analyte of interest. This may, however, be overcome through improved modern cleanup techniques that remove impurities [12].

6.1.2 High-performance liquid chromatography

High-performance liquid chromatography (HPLC) is now most commonly used for mycotoxin determination offering good sensitivity and precision, coupled with ease of automation [12, 19]. After extraction and cleanup, samples are injected into the HPLC column, individual compounds are separated based on their affinity for the column matrix and the mobile phase solvent [27]. To enhance fluorescence for better mycotoxin quantification using the HPLC-FLD technique, derivatization is important [12]. Pre-column derivatization with trifluoroacetic acid (TFA), or post-column derivatization, with bromine or iodine, can be used to identify aflatoxins [17]. Photochemical post-column derivatization may provide a cheaper alternative, whereas specific cyclodextrins may be incorporated in the mobile phase for non-chemical enhancement of fluorescence [28]. Despite offering good sensitivity and specificity, HPLC-FLD techniques are limited by expensive equipment requiring operation by experienced staff and may require laborious sample preparation procedures [12, 19].

Recent utilization of ultra-HPLC (UHPLC) methods that are based upon increasing the mobile phase pumping pressure up to 1000 bar and above and reduction of particle size from 5 μm (HPLC) to 1–2 μm (UHPLC) improves resolution, sensitivity, and achieves rapid chromatographic separation as a result of increased speed and resolution between analytes [39, 40]. However, to avoid the high cost of the UHPLC system, columns packed with materials having solid core particles, coated with an outer layer of porous material can achieve more efficient separations at a much faster rate than with standard columns eliminating the need for expensive high-pressure facility because they are able to work at standard pressures (up to 600 bar) and can be used on all HPLC systems [41].

6.1.3 Liquid chromatography/mass spectrometry

Liquid chromatography with mass spectrometry (LC/MS) is a technique that allows more sensitive and selective determination of multiple mycotoxins in complex matrices with improved limits of detection and quantification [27]. Atmospheric pressure chemical ionization (APCI), atmospheric pressure photo ionization (APPI), and electrospray ionization (ESI) interfaces are currently employed in modern LC/MS instrumentation owing to their robustness, easy handling, high sensitivity, accuracy, and analyte selectivity and compatibility to a wide range of compound polarities [22, 42].

Liquid chromatography coupled to high-resolution mass spectrometry (LC-HRMS) equipment has been developed that can significantly increase the sensitivity and specificity of multi-mycotoxin assays [37].

Liquid chromatography with tandem mass spectrometry (LC-MS/MS) has been increasingly used to provide a simultaneous determination of different classes of mycotoxins, including the regulated mycotoxins, thus affording to increase sample throughput and decreasing the cost per analysis [11]. However, given the complexity of matrixes to be analyzed and the wide-ranging physical and chemical mycotoxin properties, such methods require great skill to develop [11, 22, 42].

Mass spectrometry detectors linked to HPLC, UHPLC, and GC systems can increase their separation and identification power. However, the MS facilities are expensive with complex laboratory requirements, require skilled operators, and may suffer solvent limitations [23].

6.1.4 Gas chromatography

Gas chromatography (GC) may be used to determine mycotoxins that are volatile within the column [19]. For example, GC coupled with electron capture detection (ECD), flame ionization detection (FID) or mass spectrometric detection (MS) may be used for trichothecene or patulin determination. However, when compared to alternative methods, GC requires prior cleanup of extracts and pre-column derivatization to increase the volatility and sensitivity of the toxins [11, 17]. Although having successful applications, GC has several disadvantages that include the analyzed sample to be volatile or converted into a volatile sample, problems with the thermal stability of the sample leading to losses, and the high cost of the equipment [23].

6.2 Rapid screening methods

Rapid screening methods, that include immunochemical techniques, varying from simple lateral flow and enzyme-linked immunosorbent assays (ELISA) to highly sophisticated immunosensors, are based upon binding of an antigen, for example a mycotoxin to a specific antibody, and often do not require any cleanup or analyte enrichment steps [11, 18, 43].

6.2.1 ELISA techniques

The enzyme-linked immunosorbent assay (ELISA) technique utilizes a specific antibody to bind the target molecule directly or conjugated with the enzyme and interaction with a chromogenic substrate to give a measurable result [18, 23]. However, due to the low molecular weight of mycotoxins, they are not immunogenic and must be conjugated to a carrier molecule to achieve immunogenicity. The ELISA technique can be highly sensitive and specific, portable, rapid, and simple to use with high sample turnover. However, ELISA has a number of disadvantages that include single-use kits that can increase the cost of bulk screening, high matrix dependence, cross-reactivity, and limited detection range due to the narrow sensitivity of the antibodies [13, 23].

6.2.2 Immunosensor/biosensor techniques

Biosensors are based upon the interaction of a mycotoxin with a recognition system fabricated as a layer onto the surface of a matrix substance that induces a change that is converted into a measurable electronic signal by a transducer. This provides great sensitivity and selectivity, easy application, low cost, and portability [27, 44]. Biosensors are often classified by the type of toxin-binding element (e.g., antibody, aptamer, imprinted polymers, etc.) as well as by the technology used for signal transduction and detection (e.g., optical, electrochemical, piezoelectric, etc.) [33].

A number of biosensor/immunosensor assays and techniques have been developed for mycotoxin determination, including fiber optic devices, surface plasmon resonance (SPR), dip-stick and lateral flow devices, fluorescence polarization, time-resolved fluorescence, microbead, capillary electrophoresis (CE), and electrochemical and piezoelectric immunoassays [45, 46]. These techniques are outlined in the following subsections.

6.2.2.1 Optical biosensors and fiber optic devices

Optical sensors, based on a variation of optical signals generated by a transducer from molecular recognition events on a sensing element are divided into many subclasses depending on the type of signal generated, including calorimetric, fluorescent, chemiluminescent, and surface plasmon resonance [35]. Photoelectrochemical optical biosensors use light as an excitation source and photocurrent as the recognition signal, whereas another subset of optical biosensors uses total internal reflection ellipsometry with localized surface plasmon resonance for detection with an optical planar waveguide polarization interferometer [33]. For example, fluorescent-based fiber optic devices can capture fluorescence emission from the fluorescently labeled mycotoxin or the naturally fluorescent mycotoxin, for example, aflatoxin when they bind to the fiber optic surface and transmit it to a sensitive detector [45]. A commercial device “Octet” based on biolayer interferometry to detect changes in the interference pattern of light reflected from the surface of optical fiber when materials bind to the tip of the fiber has been developed and available from ForteBio (Menlo Park, Calif., USA) [47, 48].

6.2.2.2 Surface plasmon resonance

The SPR technique is based upon the property that the binding of materials to a surface, for example, the binding of antibodies to the mycotoxin, can alter the refractive index near that surface. The SPR device measures the small changes in the angle, or intensity, of internally reflected light that results from the binding event, and the magnitude of the response is influenced by the amount of material adhering to the surface. Alternatively, surface plasmons may be used to excite fluorophores captured on a surface, a technique is known as surface plasmon-enhanced fluorescence spectroscopy (SPFS). With this technique, light is used to excite plasmons (electron charge density waves) in a thin film of gold foil attached to the surface of a glass prism, the resonance of which enhances the fluorescence of the captured fluorophores, for example, the labeled antibody [45, 46, 49]. Using imaging, SPR (iSPR) allows multiple binding events on different regions of the sensor surface to be monitored simultaneously (multiplexing), hence capable of measuring multiple antigen-antibody interactions simultaneously in a single injection [49, 50].

The advantages of SPR include rapid and simple cleanup procedures, short analysis times, reusable sensor chips, and not necessarily requiring competition or labeled reagents for detection. It has great potential for multiplexing, with a wide variety of commercially available devices [46, 49]. However, like most immunoassays, SPR can be influenced by matrix effects that can be dealt with by increasing the dilution of the sample extract or by cleanup of the extract before the detection step [46].

6.2.2.3 Lateral flow devices

Lateral flow strip and dipstick devices (immunochromatographic test devices) use rapid disposable devices that may be attached with the toxin or the antibody that can bear enzymatic, liposome associated, or colloidal gold labels to detect the presence of mycotoxins [45]. Colloidal gold is frequently used as a label in test strips developed for mycotoxins due to availability, ease of production, and ease of conjugate formation with antibodies [51]. "Mycotoxin in the sample extract interacts with colloidal gold conjugated anti-mycotoxin antibodies at the base of the stick, with both bound and unbound antibodies moving along the stick membrane, passing a test line composed of immobilized mycotoxin, which will bind free antibody to form a visible line indicating a level of aflatoxin contamination below the test cut-off value. The control line further along the stick is composed of anti-antibodies to ensure complete extract migration along the strip" [28].

The related, membrane-based flow-through device, also known as enzyme-linked immunofiltration assay (ELIFA) differs from lateral flow devices, in that the applied liquid flows perpendicularly through the membrane rather than laterally, where it is collected on an absorbent pad on the opposite side of the membrane. It uses an enzymatic label that requires a substrate-incubation step, with the test and control lines being generated by an enzyme-substrate color reaction [28, 45].

Because of their easy application, efforts to develop dipstick and lateral flow assays for mycotoxins are likely to continue, particularly using stable, nonenzymatic labels [45], with a number of devices already being commercially available [17]. Also, innovative labels based on nanoparticle applications, such as quantum dots (QDs), gold nanoparticles (AuNPs), magnetic nanoparticles (Fe_3O_4), carbon nanoparticles (CNPs), time-resolved fluorescent microspheres (TRFM), have been developed for signal amplification in LFD, which can improve detection. Moreover, the advent of a fluorescence quenching principle in lateral flow immunoassays (LFIA) in contrast to traditional competitive LFIA increases the sensitivity of the LFIA [35, 52].

6.2.2.4 Fluorescence polarization and time-resolved fluorescence

Fluorescence polarization (FP) immunoassays are solution-phase assays that rely on the measurement of change in the rate of rotation of a fluorescent-labeled mycotoxin (tracer) when it forms an immune complex with the added antitoxin antibody after competing with unlabeled mycotoxin in the sample extract [28, 45, 46]. FP can be used to measure the rate of association of the toxin with the antibody (kinetic assays) or the equilibrium point in a competition reaction (equilibrium assays). Critically, FP relies on the proper selection of antibody and tracer pairs [45, 46].

Unlike FP immunoassays, time-resolved fluorescent immunoassays (TR-FIA) use the property of fluorescence lifetime to measure the rate of decay of a fluorophore that is associated with a mycotoxin [45]. The newer fluorescent materials known as lanthanides, such as Eu (III) and Tb (III), have much longer fluorescence lifetimes that can eliminate the background fluorescence interference from the matrix, thus improving the sensitivity of methods based on TR-FIA [35].

The fact that FP is a homogeneous assay that does not require the separation of the free and bound tracer, may eliminate additional steps, such as washing, in competitive ELISA, thus increasing method rapidity [53]. However, like most immunoassays, it can be affected by the presence of a matrix, which can be controlled through dilution, cleanup, matrix-matched calibration curves, or data normalization [46, 53]. Although the available FP immunoassay readers are not capable of multi-mycotoxin detection, the potential speed of FP assays combined with the portability of the devices, suggests this technology has a promising future [46].

6.2.2.5 Microbead assays

Microbead assays use antibodies or antigens attached to the microbeads in miniaturized IAC assays, often with the cleanup and detection steps performed on a single instrument. It can be affected by poor re-usability of the columns due to fouling and reduced functional capacity of antibodies [45].

6.2.2.6 Capillary electrophoretic immunoassays

Capillary electrophoresis (CE) employs capillaries that are injected with the cleaned sample extracts in aqueous buffer solutions where they are separated in an electrical field before detection, typically using fluorescence or UV absorbance [23, 45]. The CE methods have comparable sensitivity, precision, and accuracy to HPLC methods, use less expensive capillaries, eliminate the use of organic solvents and take shorter analysis times, thus making them viable alternatives to HPLC [17].

6.2.2.7 Electrochemical immunosensor assays

Electrochemical immunosensors for mycotoxin determination are based on the high-affinity interaction between antigen and specific antibodies that can be transformed into a measured electrochemical signal based on a variety of electrochemical techniques [54]. They can be categorized into amperometric, potentiometric, conductometric, impedimetric, and voltammetric sensors according to the types of detectable electrical signals [35]. In their simplest format, the immobilized antibody is bound to the surface of a screen-printed electrode, and the final enzymatic stage develops a reaction product that can be measured by its electrical properties [28].

These electrochemical assays can be affected by factors that influence the interface between antigen and antibody, including solvent-matrix interactions and the reduction/oxidation potential of the diluent. The extent of testing using this technology, the accessibility of components, and the capacity for miniaturization, suggest future utility of these devices in the detection of aflatoxins [46].

6.2.2.8 Piezoelectric sensors

Piezoelectric sensors often called quartz crystal microbalance (QCM) are based upon piezoelectric quartz crystals and they work through the application of an alternating current to a quartz crystal, which induces oscillations of the crystal, the frequency of which depends in part on the thickness of the crystal, for example, after mycotoxin binding on immobilized antibodies [46]. Mass change on the sensory layer of the surface of the gold-plated crystal quartz transducer causes specific measurable vibrations of the crystal in response to an electrical signal [20]. The advantage of QCM is that they do not require the use of labeled reagents [46].

In general terms, immunochemical techniques are affected by high matrix dependence, cross-reactivity, and loss of antibody stability under the extreme environment, such as pH, organic solvents, and high temperature. Moreover, the cost of their development may be high and requires a stable source of antibodies to ensure continuity of analytical performance and stability. Therefore, the development of synthetic receptors can solve some of these challenges, particularly, problems associated with antibody stability in an extreme environment [18, 44, 54]. As an example, [55] developed an aptamer-based assay for the detection of AFB_1 in corn samples that exhibited a wide dynamic range from 0.1 to 10 ng/mL, limit of detection of 0.11 ng/mL, and recovery values between 60.4 and 105.5% that were described as promising results.

It is worthy to note that, chemical and biochemical sensor devices are increasingly developed based on advanced microchip technology, including microfluidic chips and microarrays for portability, easy on-site field application, robustness, reliability, reduced cost, rapidity, high throughput, and increased sensitivity. Also, the advent of innovative labels based on nanoparticle application has led to a significant improvement in their detection capability. Examples of these include the microfluidic devices based on flow-through (capillary electromigration) and lateral flow formats and the emerging microchip-based sensing methods, such as surface plasmon resonance (SPR) and magnet nonotag-based detection [35, 56, 57].

6.3 Noninvasive techniques

Noninvasive techniques, such as spectroscopic and imaging techniques [27], DNA microarrays, electronic chemical sensors (electronic nose and tongue), and polymerase chain reaction-based methods [27, 44] provide a potential approach for rapid nondestructive detection of fungal infection and mycotoxin contamination on grains. However, many of these techniques may either be expensive and/or may need further validation studies.

7. Conclusions and analysis in resource-limited settings

All components of the food supply chain can become contaminated with aflatoxins and other mycotoxins. For food to meet safety standards, and for the development of mitigation strategies, determination of the degree of contamination is required. Analytical procedures for aflatoxin detection and quantification remain central to resolving this important food and feed safety issues. The many issues surrounding robust mycotoxin analysis have been addressed in a number of books [58–61] that the interested reader may wish to consult.

Since the discovery of aflatoxins, there has been a huge international effort to develop appropriate analytical procedures. However, all techniques have had to overcome a number of significant problems, including:

1. Diverse chemical structures that require individual methods for different mycotoxins;

2. Separation of structurally similar compounds;

3. Mycotoxins occur in very low concentrations in different commodities, thus removal or cleanup of the food/feed matrix is required. Each commodity may require a different cleanup procedure;

4. Due to the uneven distribution of mycotoxins in a commodity, it is important to analyze many samples that have been collected using a validated sampling plan.

As is apparent in this chapter, there are a plethora of approaches, both quantitative and qualitative, for aflatoxin analysis that overcame these problems. The advantages and disadvantages of the different analytical approaches are listed in Appendix 1 and examples of biosensor platforms for mycotoxin detection and their performance in terms of limit of detection is given in Appendix 2. Although, the conventional analytical techniques, particularly HPLC linked to the mass spectrometer or fluorescent detectors are indispensable to confirm the quantities of contamination and for determining the chemical identity of the various groups of mycotoxins, equipment is very expensive and there are ongoing instrument maintenance and solvent costs, and specially trained analysts are required. However, these techniques do not apply to resource-limited settings. The initial technique used for aflatoxin analysis was TLC, and it is still used in many laboratories, especially in developing countries, as it does not require expensive laboratory equipment.

The development of screening methods that provide rapid, low-cost analysis of large number of samples is required for food surveillance, particularly in low-income countries. For the most part, screening methods are specific, sensitive, and relatively simple to operate. There is also a need in low-income rural communities for rapid screening methods, where an electrical supply is often unavailable [62]. ELISAs and dipstick/lateral flow devices are simple to operate and are used widely in developing countries. However, before use, operators need to be confident that the assay kit is "fit for purpose," and is appropriate for the commodity matrix to be tested [62]. If the assay kit is not valid for the commodity tested, cross-reactivity may occur and the number of the false positive sample will increase. There are increasing efforts to develop multi-toxin screening assays, as aflatoxin is often found in association with other mycotoxins, including fumonisins and deoxynivalenol [6]. This information is important, as it is essential to know the extent of toxin exposure so the appropriate public health and mitigation steps can be undertaken. Finally, it is very important that the results obtained in the field with rapid screening tests give comparable results to quantitative analysis in regulatory laboratories.

Appendix

Appendix 1.

Advantages and disadvantages of conventional mycotoxin analytical techniques.

Method	Advantages	Disadvantages
TLC	Simple, inexpensive, and rapid Can be used for screening Simultaneous analysis of multiple mycotoxins Sensitive for aflatoxins and ochratoxin A	Poor sensitivity (for some mycotoxins) Poor precision Separation may require two-dimensional analysis Quantitative when used with a densitometer
GC	Simultaneous analysis of multiple mycotoxins Good sensitivity May be automated (autosampler) Provides confirmation (MS detector)	Expensive equipment Specialist expertise required Derivatization required Matrix interference problems Nonlinear calibration curve Drifting response Carry-over effects from previous sample Variation in reproducibility & repeatability
HPLC	Good sensitivity Good selectivity Good repeatability May be automated (autosampler) Short analysis times Official methods available	Expensive equipment Specialist expertise required May require derivatization
LC/MS	Simultaneous analysis of multiple mycotoxins Good sensitivity (LC/MS/MS) Provides confirmation No derivatization required	Very expensive equipment Specialist expertise requested Sensitivity relies on ionization technique Matrix-assisted calibration curve (for quantitative analysis)
ELISA	Simple sample preparation Inexpensive equipment High sensitivity Simultaneous analysis of multiple samples Suitable for screening Limited use of organic solvents Visual assessment	Cross-reactivity with related mycotoxins Matrix interference problems Possible false positive/negative results Confirmatory LC analysis required Critical quantitation near regulatory limits Semi-quantitative (visual assessment)
Rapid tests	Simple and fast (5–10 min) No expensive equipment required Limited use of organic solvents Suitable for screening purposes Can be used *in situ*	Qualitative or semi-quantitative (cut-off level) Possible false positive/negative results Cross-reactivity with related mycotoxins Matrix interference problems Lack of sensitivity near regulatory limits

TLC - Thin Layer Chromatography, GC - Gas Chromatography, HPLC - High-Performance Liquid Chromatography, LC/MS - Liquid Chromatography with Mass Spectrometry, LC/MS/MS - Liquid Chromatography with tandem Mass Spectrometry, MS - Mass Spectrometer, ELISA - Enzyme-linked Immunosorbent Assay.
Adapted from reference [17].

Appendix 2.

Examples of biosensor platforms for mycotoxin detection.

Target	Principle	Signal material	Sample	LOD
FB1/ DON	Competitive LFIA	gold nanospheres/gold nanoflowers	Grain	20/5 ng/mL
DON/ AFB1	Competitive fluorescent LFIA	α-Fe_2O_3 nanocubes	Food	0.18/0.01 ng/mL
ZEN/ OTA/ FB1	Competitive fluorescent LFIA	Quantum dot nanobeads	Wheat	5/20/10 ng/mL
AFB1/ ZEN	Competitive fluorescent LFIA	Time-resolved fluorescence microspheres	Maize	0.05/0.07 ng/mL
DON/T-2/ZEN	Competitive fluorescent LFIA	Amorphous carbon nanoparticles	Maize	20/13/1 μg/kg
OTA/ AFB1	Optical (calorimetric)	Aptamer, magnetic nanoparticles/graphene oxide, and magnetic nanoparticles@gold	Agricultural products	0.5/5 ng/mL
AFB1/ AFG1	Optical (calorimetric)	Gold and silver nanoparticles	Pistachio, wheat, coffee, milk	2.7/7.3 ng/mL
AFB1/ OTA/ FB1	Optical (fluorescent protein microarray)	Antibody, TiO2-modified porous silicon	Rice, maize, wheat	0.093 ng/mL
AFB1/ FB1	Optical (fluorescent)	Aptamer, graphene oxide/magnetic nanoparticles, and CdTe quantum dots	Peanut	6.2/16.2 pg/mL
FB1/ OTA	Optical (fluorescent)	Aptamer, time-resolved nanoparticles, and magnetic nanoparticles	Maize	0.015 pg/mL
AFB1	Optical (fluorescent quenching)	Aptamer, CdZnTe quantum dots, and gold nanoparticles	Peanut	20 pg/mL
AFB1/ OTA	Optical (Chemiluminescence)	Antibody and silver nanoparticles	Red yeast rice	0.44/0.83 pg/ mL
AFB1	Optical (SPR)	Antibody, gold chips	Grains	2.51 ppb
AFB1	Optical (SPR)	Antibody, gold nanoparticles, and self-assembled monolayer gold chips	Wheat	0.003 nmol/L
AFB1	Electrochemical (impedimetric)	Cysteine/carbon nanotubes-modified gold electrode immunosensor	Maize flour	0.79 pg/g
ZEN	Electrochemical (differential pulse voltammetry)	Screen-printed electrode immunosensor	Beer and wine	0.25 ng/mL

Target	Principle	Signal material	Sample	LOD
AFB1	Electrochemical (cyclic voltammetry)	Graphene quantum dots and gold nanoparticles-modified indium tin oxide electrode immunosensor	Maize	0.1 ng/mL
AFB1	Electrochemical (square wave voltammetry)	Gold electrode aptasensor	Beer	2nmol/L

FB1 - Fumonisin B1, DON - Deoxynivalenol, ZEN - Zearalenone, AFB1 - Aflatoxin B1, AFG1 - Aflatoxin G1, T-2 - T-2 toxin, OTA - Ochratoxin A, LFIA - Lateral Flow Immunoassay, SPR - Surface Plasmon Resonance, LOD - Limit of Detection.
Adapted from reference [35].

Author details

Godfrey Z. Magoke[1*], Robyn G. Alders[2,3,4], Mark Krockenberger[5] and Wayne L. Bryden[6]

1 Tanzania Veterinary Laboratory Agency, Dar es Salaam, Tanzania

2 Global Health Programme, Chatham House, UK

3 Kyeema Foundation, Brisbane, Australia

4 Development Policy Centre, Australian National University, Canberra, Australia

5 Faculty of Science, School of Veterinary Science, University of Sydney, Australia

6 University of Queensland, Brisbane, Australia

*Address all correspondence to: gmagoke@gmail.com

References

[1] Wu F, Stacy SL, Kensler TW. Global risk assessment of aflatoxins in maize and peanuts: Are regulatory standards adequately and protective? Toxicological Sciences. 2013;**135**(1):251-259

[2] Bryden WL. Mycotoxins in the food chain and human health implications. In: Nriagu J, editor. Encyclopedia of Environmental Health. 2nd ed. USA: Elsevier Inc; 2019. pp. 515-523

[3] Richard JL. Discovery of aflatoxins and significant historical features. Toxin Reviews. 2008;**27**:171-201

[4] Kensler TW, Roebuck BD, Wogan GN, Groopman JD. Aflatoxin: A 50 year odyssey of mechanistic and translational toxicology. Toxicological Sciences. 2011;**120**:28-48. DOI: 10.1093/toxsci/kfq283

[5] Bryden WL. Mycotoxin contamination of the feed supply chain: Implications for animal productivity and feed security. Animal Feed Science and Technology. 2012;**173**:134-158

[6] Gruber-Dorninger C, Jenkins T, Schatzmayr G. Global mycotoxin occurrence in feed: A ten-year survey. Toxins. 2019;**11**:375

[7] Eskola M, Kos G, Elliott CT, Hajšlová J, Sultan Mayar S, Krska R. Worldwide contamination of food-crops with mycotoxins: Validity of the widely cited 'FAO estimate' of 25%. Critical Reviews in Food Science and Nutrition. 2020;**60**:2773

[8] Williams JH, Phillips TD, Jolly PE, Stiles JK, Jolly CM, Aggarwal D. Human aflatoxicosis in developing countries: A review of toxicology, exposure, potential health consequences, and interventions. The American Journal of Clinical Nutrition. 2004;**80**:1106

[9] Strosnider H, Azziz-Baumgartner E, Banziger M, Bhat RV, Breiman R, Brune M, et al. Workgroup report: Public health strategies for reducing aflatoxin exposure in developing countries. Environmental Health Perspective. 2020;**114**:1898

[10] Wild CP, Gong YY. Mycotoxins and human disease: A largely ignored global health issue. Carcinogenesis. 2010;**31**:71

[11] Krska R, Schubert P, Molinelli A, Sulyok M, Macdonald S, Crews C. Mycotoxin analysis: An update. Food Additives and Contaminants. 2008; **25**(2):152-163

[12] Gilbert J, Anklam E. Validation of analytical methods for determining mycotoxins in foodstuffs. Trends in Analytical Chemistry. 2002;**21**(6-7): 468-486

[13] Krska R, Welzig E, Berthiller F, Molinelli A, Mizaikoff B. Advances in the analysis of mycotoxins and its quality assurance. Food Additives and Contaminants. 2005;**22**(4):345-353

[14] Whitaker TB. Sampling for mycotoxins. In: Magan N, Olsen M, editors. Mycotoxins in Food. UK: Woodhead Publishing; 2004. pp. 69-87

[15] Whitaker TB. Sampling foods for mycotoxins. Food Additives and Contaminants. 2006;**23**:50-61. DOI: 10.1080/02652030500241587

[16] Pereira VL, Fernandes JO, Cunha SC. Mycotoxins in cereals and related foodstuffs: A review on occurrence and recent methods of analysis. Trends in

Food Science & Technology. 2014;**36**: 96-163

[17] Pascale M, Visconti A. Overview of detection methods for mycotoxins. In: Leslie JF, Bandyopadhyay R, Visconti A, editors. Mycotoxins Detection Methods, Management, Public Health and Agricultural Trade. Cambridge (MA): CABI International; 2008. pp. 171-183

[18] Turner NW, Bramhmbhatt H, Szabo-Vezse M, Poma A, Coker R, Piletsky SA. Analytical methods for determination of mycotoxins: An update (2009–2014). AnalyticaChimicaActa. 2015;**901**:12-33

[19] Rahmani A, Jinap S, Soleimany F. Qualitative and quantitative analysis of mycotoxins. Comprehensive Reviews in Food Science and Food Safety. 2009;**8**: 202-251

[20] Agriopoulou S, Stamatelopoulou E, Varzakas T. Advances in analysis and detection of major mycotoxins in foods. Foods. 2020;**9**:518

[21] Bertuzzi T, Rastelli S, Mulazzi A, Pietri A. Evaluation and Improvement of Extraction Methods for the Analysis of Aflatoxins B-1, B-2, G (1) and G (2) from Naturally Contaminated Maize. Food Analytical Methods. 2012;**5**:512-519

[22] Zoellner P, Mayer-Helm B. Trace mycotoxin analysis in complex biological and food matrices by liquid chromatography-atmospheric pressure ionisation mass spectrometry. Journal of Chromatography. A. 2006;**1136**: 123-169

[23] Turner NW, Subrahmanyam S, Piletsky SA. Analytical methods for determination of mycotoxins: A review. Analytica Chimica Acta. 2009;**632**(2): 168-180

[24] Yiantzi E, Psillakis E, Tyrovola K, Kalogerakis N. Vortex-assisted liquid-liquid microextraction of octylphenol, nonylphenol and bisphenol-A. Talanta. 2010;**80**:2057-2062

[25] Abu-Bakar NB, Makahleh A, Saad B. Vortex-assisted liquid-liquid microextraction coupled with high performance liquid chromatography for the determination of furfurals and patulin in fruit juices. Talanta. 2014;**120**: 47-54

[26] Papadopoulou A, Roman IP, Canals A, Tyrovola K, Psillakis E. Fast screening of perfluorooctanesulfonate in water using vortex-assisted liquid-liquid microextraction coupled to liquid chromatography-mass spectrometry. AnalyticaChimicaActa. 2011;**691**:56-61

[27] Yao H, Hruska Z, Mavungu DJ. Developments in detection and determination of aflatoxins. World Mycotoxin Journal. 2015;**8**(2):181-191

[28] Shephard GS. Aflatoxin analysis at the beginning of the twenty-first century: A review. Analytical Bioanalytical Chemistry. 2009;**395**(5): 1215-1224

[29] Capriotti AL, Cavaliere C, Lagana A, Piovesana S, Samperi R. Recent trends in matrix solid-phase dispersion. Trac-Trends in Analytical Chemistry. 2013;**43**: 53-66

[30] Khayoon WS, Saad B, Salleh B, Manaf NHA, Latiff AA. Micro-solid phase extraction with liquid chromatography-tandem mass spectrometry for the determination of aflatoxins in coffee and malt beverage. Food Chemistry. 2014;**147**:287-294

[31] Hashemi M, Taherimaslak Z, Rashidi S. Application of magnetic solid

phase extraction for separation and determination of aflatoxins B-1 and B-2 in cereal products by high performance liquid chromatography-fluorescence detection. Journal of Chromatography. B, Analytical Technologies in the Biomedical and Life Sciences. 2014a; **960**:200-208

[32] Hashemi M, Taherimaslak Z, Rashidi S. Enhanced spectrofluorimetric determination of aflatoxin M-1 in liquid milk after magnetic solid phase extraction. SpectrochimicaActa Part A-Molecular and Biomolecular Spectroscopy. 2014b;**128**:583-590

[33] Tittlemier SA, Brunkhorst J, Cramer B, DeRosa MC, Lattanzio VMT, Malone R, et al. Sumarah MW. Developments in mycotoxin analysis: An update for 2019-2020. World Mycotoxin Journal. 2021;**14**(1):3-26

[34] Lucci P, Derrien D, Alix F, Perollier C, Bayoudh S. Molecularly imprinted polymer solid-phase extraction for detection of zearalenone in cereal sample extracts. Analytica Chimica Acta. 2010;**672**:15-19

[35] Li R, Wen Y, Wang F, He P. Recent advances in immunoassays and biosensors for mycotoxins detection in feedstuffs and foods. Journal of Animal Science and Biotechnology. 2021;**12**:108

[36] Nunez O, Gallart-Ayala H, Martins CPB, Lucci P. New trends in fast liquid chromatography for food and environmental analysis. Journal of Chromatography A. 2012;**1228**:298

[37] Berthiller F, Burdaspal PA, Crews C, Iha MH, Krska R, Lattanzio VMT, et al. Developments in mycotoxin analysis: An update for 2012–2013. World Mycotoxin Journal. 2014;7:3-33

[38] Berthiller F, Brera C, Crews C, Iha MH, Krska R, Lattanzio VMT, et al. Developments in mycotoxin analysis: An update for 2013–2014. World Mycotoxin Journal. 2015;**8**(1):5-36

[39] Li P, Zhang Z, Hu X, Zhang Q. Advanced hyphenated chromatographic-mass spectrometry in mycotoxin determination: Current status and prospects. Mass Spectrometry Reviews. 2013;**32**:420-452

[40] O'Mahony J, Clarke L, Whelan M, O'Kennedy R, Lehotay SJ, Danaher M. The use of ultra-high pressure liquid chromatography with tandem mass spectrometric detection in the analysis of agrochemical residues and mycotoxinsin food – Challenges and applications. Journal of Chromatography A. 2013; **1292**:83-95

[41] Medina A, Magan N. Comparison of three different C-18 HPLC columns with different particle sizes for the optimization of aflatoxins analysis. Journal of Chromatography. B, Analytical Technologies in the Biomedical and Life Sciences. 2012;**889**: 138-143

[42] Songsermsakul P, Razzazi-Fazeli E. A Review of recent trends in applications of Liquid Chromatography – Mass Spectrometry for determination of mycotoxins. Journal of Liquid Chromatography and Related Technologies. 2008;**31**:1641-1686

[43] Zheng MZ, Richard JL, Binder J. A review of rapid methods for the analysis of mycotoxins. Mycopathologia. 2006; **161**:261-273. DOI: 10.1007/s11046-006-0215-6

[44] Logrieco A, Arrigan DWM, Brengel-Pesce K, Siciliano P, Tothill I. DNA arrays, electronic noses and tongues, biosensors and receptors for rapid

detection of toxigenic fungi and mycotoxins: A review. Food Additives and Contaminants. 2005;**22**: 335-344

[45] Maragos CM. Emerging technologies for mycotoxin detection. Journal of Toxicology-Toxin Reviews. 2004; **23**(2–3):317-344

[46] Maragos CM, Busman M. Rapid and advanced tools for mycotoxin analysis: A review. Food Additives and Contaminants Part A-Chemistry Analysis Control Exposure & Risk Assessment. 2010;**27**(5): 688-700

[47] Maragos CM. Detection of deoxynivalenol using biolayer interferometry. Mycotoxin Research. 2011;**27**:157-165

[48] Maragos CM. Signal amplification using colloidal gold in a biolayer interferometry-based immunosensor for the mycotoxindeoxynivalenol. Food Additives & Contaminants. Part A, Chemistry, Analysis, Control, Exposure& Risk Assessment. 2012;**29**: 1108

[49] Hossain MZ, Mccormick SP, Maragos CM. An Imaging Surface Plasmon Resonance biosensor assay for the detection of T-2 toxin and masked T-2 toxin-3-glucoside in wheat. Toxins. 2018;**2018**:10

[50] Hossain MZ, Maragos CM. Gold nanoparticle-enhanced multiplexed imaging surface plasmon resonance (iSPR) detection of fusariummycotoxins in wheat. Biosensors & Bioelectronics. 2018;**101**:245-252

[51] Krska R, Molinelli A. Rapid test strips for analysis of mycotoxins in food and feed. Analytical and Bioanalytical Chemistry. 2009;**393**:67-71

[52] Oliveira IS, da Silva Junior AG, de Andrade CAS, Oliveira MDL. Biosensors for early detection of fungi spoilage and toxigenic and mycotoxins in food. Current Opinion in Food Science. 2019; **29**:64-79

[53] Maragos C. Fluorescence polarization immunoassay of mycotoxins. a review. Toxins. 2009;**1**: 196-207

[54] Vidal JC, Bonel L, Ezquerra A, Hernandez S, Bertolin JR, Cubel C, et al. Electrochemical affinity biosensors for detection of mycotoxins: A review. Biosensors & Bioelectronics. 2013;**49**: 146-158

[55] Shim WB, Mun H, Joung HA, Ofori JA, Chung DH, Kim MG. Chemiluminescence competitive aptamer assay for the detection of aflatoxin B_1 in corn samples. Food Control. 2014;**36**(1):30-35

[56] Li P, Zhang Z, Zhang Q, Zhang N, Zhang W, Ding X, et al. Current development of microfluidic immunosensing approaches for mycotoxin detection via capillary electromigration and lateral flow technology. Electrophoresis. 2012; **33**(15):2253-2265

[57] Zhang Z, Yu L, Xu L, Hu X, Li P, Zhang Q, et al. Biotoxin sensing in food and environment via microchip. Electrophoresis. 2014;**35**(11):1547-1559

[58] Cole RJ. Modern Methods in the Analysis and Structural Elucidation of Mycotoxins. New York: Academic Press; 1986

[59] Trucksess MW, Pohland AE. Methods in Molecular Biology. Totowa, NJ: Mycotoxin Protocols Humana Press Inc; 2001

[60] Magan N, Olsen M. Mycotoxins in Food: Detection and Control. UK: Woodhead Publishing; 2004

[61] De Saeger S. editor. Determining Mycotoxins and Mycotoxigenic Fungi in Food and Feed. Woodhead Publishing, UK; 2011

[62] Shephard GS. Mycotoxin crises: Fit-for-purpose analytical responses in the developing world. Journal of AOAC International. 2018;**101**:609-612

Chapter 6

Review of QuEChERS Methods for the Analysis of Mycotoxins in Food Samples

Lukman Bola Abdulra'uf, Kikelomo Elizabeth Ayeni, Abdulrahman Ibraheem, Aisha Ishaq, Abibat Monisola Junaid, Mutiat Aliu, Abubakar Lawal and Guan Huat Tan

Abstract

Mycotoxins are secondary metabolites present in foods which can cause adverse effects on humans and animals. Therefore, developing a simple, effective, sensitive and validated analytical method to monitor mycotoxins is essential. Sample preparation is an important step in the analysis of mycotoxins and other contaminants from complex food matrices. Food industries in developed and developing countries have faced serious challenges with contamination of mycotoxins especially aflatoxin in food and feed products. Thus, corn and cereal-based foods are mostly affected right from pre and postharvest periods. Owing to the complexity and structural nature of mycotoxins in foods and feeds there is an urgent need for simple, effective and environmentally friendly methods of sample preparation for the detection and quantification of aflatoxins in food samples. The paper reviews the application of the Quick, Easy, Cheap, Effective, Rugged and Safe (QuEChERS) method for the analysis of aflatoxins in foods.

Keywords: aflatoxins, chromatographic analysis, GC/MS, LC/MS, QuEChERS, sample preparation

1. Introduction

Aflatoxins are a group of chemically similar poisonous, carcinogenic fungal secondary metabolites produced by *Aspergillus flavus*, *A. parasiticus* and *A. nomius*, which are abundant in warm and humid regions of the world. They are probably the most intensively researched toxins in the world due to their carcinogenic and mutagenic effects. Aflatoxins have also been identified as a potential biological weapon for food and water contamination. The word aflatoxins is the combination of three words: first letter "A" from genus *Aspergillus*, next three letters "FLA" from species *flavus*, and the noun "TOXIN". Aflatoxins are quite stable and are resistant to degradation [1, 2]. There are about 18 different aflatoxins, and six types have been identified to be more important and they are labeled AFB1, AFB2, AFG1, AFG2, AFM1 and AFM2, and they exhibit different molecular structures. The B-group have cyclopentane ring and exhibits blue fluorescence under UV light, while the G group contains lactone ring and exhibits yellow-green fluorescence under UV light. Aflatoxins M1 and M2 are hydroxylated derivatives of aflatoxins B and were first isolated from milk. The behavior under UV light made them easily identified and quantified using fluorescence spectroscopy [1, 3]. The aim of this work is to review various aspects of QuEChERS techniques including its various modification for the analysis of aflatoxins in food samples.

2. Aflatoxin and its health impacts

Food industries in developed and developing countries are facing serious challenges with contamination of mycotoxins especially aflatoxin in food and feed products. The Food and Agricultural Organization (FAO) concluded that around 25% of the world's cereals are contaminated by mycotoxins including aflatoxins [4]. The most common food commodities affected by aflatoxins are cereals (corn, wheat, barley, maize, oats and rye), nuts (hazelnut, peanut and pistachio nut), dried fruits (fig), and spices (chili powder) [2]. Thus, aflatoxins are quite chemically stable and are highly resistant to degradation. Among the 18 common groups of aflatoxins, B1, B2, G1, G2, M1 and M2 are the major classes and derivatives of bifuranocoumarins. Health implications of contaminated aflatoxins in humans and animals through consumption, contact or inhalation of foodstuffs in both developed and developing countries cannot be underestimated, where billions of people are chemically exposed to uncontrolled amounts of aflatoxins, which causes disease known as aflatoxicosis [1]. Aflatoxins are toxic and fatal in poultry animals (livestock) and are carcinogenic to humans [5].

The International Agency for Research on Cancer (IARC) classified AFBI as class I human carcinogen and has a positive association between dietary aflatoxins and liver cell cancer (LCC). This was the third leading cancer death globally. Vomiting, abdominal pain, pulmonary edema, convulsions and coma. Enlargement of internal organs such as liver, kidneys and heart are common symptoms of aflatoxicosis. Different regions and countries have set maximum levels (MLs) for different mycotoxins in food. In Europe, limits of 2 ppb (for aflatoxin B1) and 4 ppb (for total aflatoxins (B1 + B2 + G1 + G2), for cereals and cereal products (including maize and maize products) for direct human consumption are in place. Likewise, MLs of 5 ppb for aflatoxin B1 and 10 ppb for total aflatoxins are set for maize to be sorted or otherwise processed physically before human consumption. The European Commission further set a method for sampling cereals and cereals products in view of the prescribed limits. The regulated limits of mycotoxins in the European region are defined in the regulation of the European Community EG-VO 1881/2006. Codex Alimentarius Commission is responsible for setting maximum limits for mycotoxins in food and feed at the global level. The Codex Commission has already adopted MLs for mycotoxins as shown below [6]:

1. A maximum level of 10 ppb for total aflatoxins in tree nuts (almonds, hazelnuts, pistachios and shelled Brazil nuts) 'ready-to-eat'.

2. ML of 15 ppb for total aflatoxins in peanuts and tree nuts destined for further processing.

3. ML of 2000 ppb for fumonisins in maize and maize flour for direct human consumption.

4. ML of 4000 ppb for fumonisins in maize for further processing.

5. ML of 2000 ppb for deoxynivalenol in raw cereal grains (wheat, maize and barley).

6. ML of 1000 ppb for deoxynivalenol in flour, semolina, meal and flakes derived from wheat, maize and barley.

7. ML of 200 ppb for deoxynivalenol in cereal-based foods for infants and young children.

3. Sampling in Aflatoxins

Aflatoxin is a subclass of mycotoxins which are strains of the fungi *Aspergilllus flavus* and *A. parasiticus* and the less common *A. nomius*. Aflatoxins B1, B2, G1, G2, M1 and M2 are the most common types of Aflatoxins, which can be grouped in two based on their chemical structure, that is difurocoumarocyclopentanone and ifurocoumarolactone [2]. However, many foods and feeds that are prone to mycotoxin contamination cannot be directly analyzed in the absence of extraction and clean-up steps [7]. Researchers have used various extraction and clean-up methods to extract aflatoxins from complex matrices [7]. Dry, wet and cryogenic grindings are common homogenization techniques in cereal-based foods, oil seeds, spices, trees nuts and peanuts, contaminated by aflatoxins. Spanjer et al. [8] successfully used dry milling to process peanut, pistachio, wheat, maize, cornflakes, raising and figs for the analysis of different mycotoxins including aflatoxins. Evaluation of homogenization is always done in terms of analytical results, coefficients of variation for different mills, sample and subsample sizes and particle size distributions [7].

The European Union defined sampling method for mycotoxins in agricultural commodities through Commission Regulation No EC401/2006, to show that sample preparation plays important role in the precision of the determination of mycotoxins. Hydrophobic mycotoxins are extracted in the presence of organic solvents, such as methanol, acetone, chloroform and acetonitrile, while polar mycotoxins are extracted in mixture of organic solvents and water [3, 9]. Studies have shown that near infrared region (NIR) (800–2500 nm) is capable of differentiating kernels containing >100 ppb or <10 ppb levels of total aflatoxins. Research conducted on 168 samples of corn collected from different parts of Italy demonstrates that FT-NIR spectroscopy is better, easier and faster to detect FB1 and FB2 in corn compared to other analytical methods such as HPLC and ELISA [10].

3.1 Sample Preparation

Sample preparation stage is the most crucial and critical step in the analysis of contaminants in complex food samples [11]. Owing to the complexity and structural nature of mycotoxins in foods and feeds there is an urgent need for simple, effective and environmentally friendly methods of sample preparation for the detection and quantification of aflatoxins in food samples [3]. The goals of sample treatment step are as follows.

i. ability to use smaller amount of sample

ii. improvement in online methods and reduce manual operations

iii. the usage of no or small volumes of organic solvent with less waste and friendly environment in order to approache green chemistry [12].

Indeed, sample preparation is of great importance in analytical procedures because its steps account for one-third of the errors generated by analytical [13]. An efficient sample preparation method provides reliable, precise and accurate results, especially when trace or ultra-trace level of analytes in complex matrices (biological and environmental) are analyzed. Low operational cost, adequate removal of matrices interference, use of small amount of solvent, limiting the number of steps and high reproducibility and recovery, high sample throughput are characteristics of good sample preparation [14].

Extraction methods based on QuEChERS (quick, easy, cheap, effective, rugged and safe) developed by Anastassiades and his co-researchers. Anastassiades et al. [15] have been widely used in analysis of mycotoxins (aflatoxin, ochratoxin A, zearalenone, fusarenon X, α and β zearalenone) due to their simplicity and effectiveness for isolating mycotoxins from complex matrices. In contrast, traditional methods of extraction such as liquid–liquid extraction and solid phase extraction use highly toxic solvents, time-consuming and large amount of sample. QuEChERS ensures minimum sample loss by limiting the number of steps, improving sample throughput, low operational cost and effective removal of matrix component interference with high productivity and recovery [14].

The extraction method (**Figure 1**) is based on microscale extraction/partitioning followed by dispersive solid phase extraction (dSPE) for cleanup [17]. The analyte is partitioned between an aqueous and an organic layer by using $MgSO_4$ and NaCl,

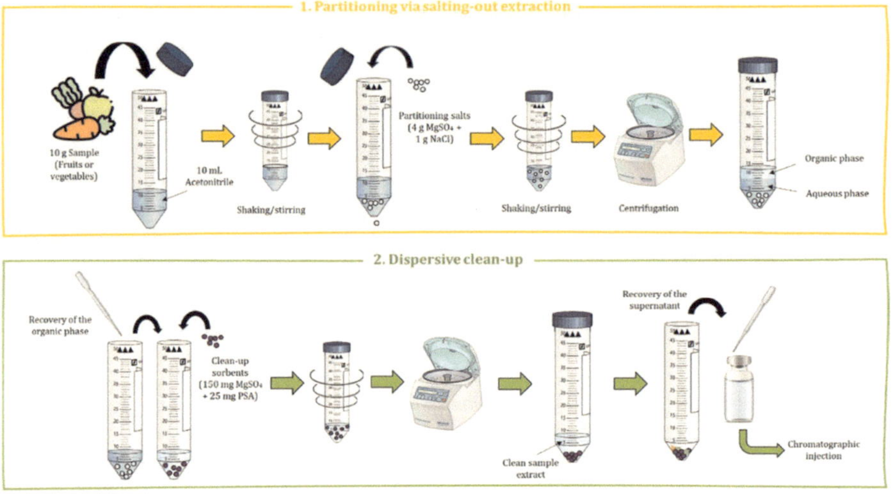

Figure 1.
Steps in original QuEChERS extraction procedure [16].

followed by manual mixing and then centrifugation for a period of time and then the supernatant is cleaned up with the combination of primary-secondary amine (PSA) adsorbent and $MgSO_4$ for the removal of interfering substances [18, 19]. The aliquot of the cleaned-up extract can then be analyzed with any of the analytical instruments.

4. Application of QuEChERS in extraction of aflatoxins

In recent times, researchers have applied QuEChERS for the analysis of aflatoxins in different food samples, although, it was initially developed for the analysis of pesticide residues [15] in fruit and vegetable samples. The different modifications of QuEChERS methods as employed in the determination of aflatoxins in food samples are hereby discussed.

Sirhan et al. [2] used QuEChERS-HPLC to detect aflatoxin in 609 samples of food consisting of 274 cereals, 87 peanuts, 78 peanut butter, 46 nuts, 46 sesame seeds; 61 Pistachio nuts, 51 seeds (sunflower, watermelon) and 51 green coffee. About 1–4 kg of each representative sample was collected and kept in dark room at 20–25°C (room temperature). A fine and homogenous powdered material was obtained through grinding and mixing processes. Factors such as solvent extraction, type and amount of drying agent, the extraction time and solvent sample ratio were optimized. All experiments were carried out using the same procedure and were tested in a blank peanut sample that had been spiked with 10.0 μg/l of aflatoxin B1 and G1 and 3.0 μg/l of aflatoxin B2 and G2. The linearity, accuracy, limit of defection (LOD), limit of quantification (LOQ), intra-day precision and inter-day precision were validated in this study. The linear concentration range from 0.059 to 30 μg/kg for aflatoxin B2 and G2 and from 0.195 to 100 mg/kg for aflatoxin B1 and G1, with correlation coefficient greater than 0.993 for all the targeted analytes The limit of detection (LOD) and limit of quantitation (LOQ) were found respectively to be 0.17 and 0.57 μg/kg in B1, 0.05 and 0.18 μg/kg in B2, 0.35 and 1.17 μg/kg in G1, and 0.06 and 0.20 μg/kg in G2. The recoveries obtained ranged between 76.3 and 98.0% with RSD values of less than 10%. The sensitivity of the method was estimated by the LOD and LOQ [2].

AFBI and AFM1 in 40 milk samples were determined simultaneously using QuEChERS with ultrahigh performance liquid chromatography coupled to quadrupole orbitrap mass spectrometry [20]. A modified QuEChERS was used to extract aflatoxin in milk. An aliquot of 10 ml sample was transferred into falcon tube containing 2.5 ml distilled water and 5.0 ml acetonitrile containing 3.35% of formic acid was then added. The mixture was vigorously vortexed for 2 min before it was subjected to ultrasonic extraction for 15 min. This was followed by addition of 4.0 g of anhydrous Na_2SO_4 and 1.2 g of NaCl, and the tube was shaken by hand for 2 min and then centrifuged for 3 min at 4000 rpm. Consequently, the supernatant was reconstituted with 500 μl of mixture of MeOH:H_2O (70:30, v/v) and filtered, then transferred for UHPLC-Q-Orbitrap HRMS analysis.

The validation and evaluation of method developed by Rodriguez-Carrasco and co-researchers were performed in accordance with SANCO (2011), by determining the linearity, matrix effect, precision, specificity and sensitivity. The recovery ranged from 75 to 91% and 81–96% for AFM1 and AFB1, respectively with RSD ranging from 7 to 16%. The linearity was found between 0.002 and 20 μg/l, with correlation coefficient R^2 greater than 0.9990. The matrix effect which was expressed as a ratio percentage between the slope of the matrix-matched calibration curve and the curve in solvent was 72 and 65% for AFB1 and AFM1, respectively. The LOQ was found to be 0.001 μg/kg and LOQ of 0.002 μg/kg, and it showed that the developed method is suitable for the determination of trace amount of aflatoxins in milk samples.

Rice samples belonging to different varieties were purchased for aflatoxins detection [21]. A modified QuEChERS method was used for the extraction of the aflatoxin from the sample. An aliquot of 3.3 g of homogenized rice was measured into a 50 ml Teflon centrifuge tube then aflatoxins were spiked at 6, 12 and 20 μg/kg concentrations. Prior to QuEChERS extraction, the spiked homogenates were stored in the dark at room temperature for 6 h to enhance absorption of aflatoxin into the sample matrix. Water (6.6 ml) and acetonitrile (10 ml) were added at 3 min intervals followed by vigorous shaking to obtain a homogenous mixture. Subsequently, 4 g of anhydrous $MgSO_4$ and 1 g of NaCl were added, shaken and centrifuged at 4000 rpm and for 5 min. The supernatant (5 ml) was transferred into another centrifuge tube containing 150 mg of PSA and 600 mg of $MgSO_4$. The mixture was shaken for 1 min and centrifuged for 5 min at 4000 rpm. The supernatant was injected into the HPLC (mobile phase containing water/methanol/acetonitrile mixture (65:25:10, v/v/v%) pumped at isocratic mode at rate of 1 ml/min, at injection volume of 20 μl. The detection was achieved at excitation and emission wavelengths of 360 and 450 nm, respectively. Validation of methods showed the limits of detection and quantification were ≤6 and ≤8 μg/kg, respectively. The linearity was between 6 and 20 μk/kg with a correlation coefficient greater than 0.99. The intra-day and inter-day recoveries were in the range 104–119% and 104–113% with RSD ≤ 12% for concentrations between 6 and 20 μg/kg.

A method, whichh was found to be sensitive, reliable, and selective was developed for the determination of 15 mycotoxins in foods and feeds using HPLC-MS with gel permeation chromatography combined with QuEChERS purification [22]. For the sample preparation, 10 g of each homogenized sample was transferred into a 100 ml centrifuge tube followed by addition of 40 ml of 84% (v/v) acetonitrile/water mixture and the mixture was homogenized for 3 min with high-speed homogenizer. The mixture was then centrifuged at 10,000 rpm for 10 min and 16 ml of the supernatant was evaporated to dryness under a stream of nitrogen at 5°C. The residue was then redissolved with 8 ml of mixture of ethyl acetate and cyclohexane (50:50 v/v) and filtered through 0.45 μm nylon filter for gel permeation chromatography (GPC) injection. A 50:50 v/v% of ethyl acetate/cyclohexane was used as the GPC mobile phase at a flow rate of 4.7 ml/min. The eluent of the GPC was collected and evaporated to dryness using rotary evaporator and the residue was redissolved with 2.5 ml acetonitrile. The redissolved residue was then vortexed with 150 mg of octadecylsilane for 1 min and an aliquot of 2 ml of the supernatant was transferred into a test tube and dried by stream of nitrogen at 50°C. The residue was then redissolved in 1 ml of methanol/10 mmol/l ammonium acetate (1:1 v/v). Finally, the solution was filtered through a 0.22 μm nylon filter and was subjected to HPLC operated at a column temperature of 35°C, with injection volume of 20 μl and mobile phase made up of solvent A (10 mmol/l ammonium acetate used for the ESI+ mode and 0.1% (v/v) aqueous ammonia used for the ESI- mode) and solvent B (methanol). The LOD of the 15 mycotoxins ranged from 0.70−5.0 μg/kg, and the recoveries ranged from 80.1−95.5% with relative standard deviation between 10.5 and 19.6%. The method gave good linear relationships and good coefficients of determination ($r^2 > 0.996$) were achieved over the concentration range of 0.5–400 ng/ml.

Miro-Abella et al. [23] used QuEChERS method followed by liquid chromatography–tandem mass spectrometry to determine 11 mycotoxins in plant-based beverages which were reported to yield 80–91% recoveries with better repeatability and reproducibility values. Limit of quantification was between 0.05 μg/l (for AFGI and AFBI) and 15 μg/l for decoxynivalenol and fumonisin B2. For the preparation of samples using QuEChERS, 50 ml centrifuge tube containing mixture of 10 ml of sample, 10 ml acetonitrile containing 1% formic acid was shaken for 1 min, then, 4 g of $MgSO_4$ and 1 g of NaCl were added to the solution and shaken vigorously for 3 min. The tubes were later centrifuged at 10,000 rpm at 20°C for 5 min. This was followed by diluting 1 ml of aliquot of organic layer as supernatant (v/v) with solvent A (water) of the mobile phase and filtered with 0.2 μm nylon filter. The linearity of the method was better with $r^2 \geq 0.993$ in all matrices and LODs were 0.001 μg/l (for AFG2, AFG1, AFB2 and AFB1), 0.04 μg/l (for FB1, FB2 and ZEA), 0.01 μg/l (for OTA and T-2), 0.1 μg/l (for DON) and 0.25 μg/l (for HT-2), with LOQs of 0.003 μg/l (for AFG2, AFG1, AFB2 and AFB1), 0.2 μg/l (for FB1, FB2 and ZEA), 0.03 μg/l (for OTA and T-2), 0.3 μg/l (for DON) and 0.9 μg/l (for HT-2). Linear range was from LOQ to 100 μg/l (for AFG2, AFG1, AFB2, AFB1 and OTA), to 500 μg/l (for DON, FB2 and T-2) and to 1000 μg/l 1 (for FB1, HT-2 and ZEA). The results of the developed method showed that QuEChERS approach was suitable for the extraction of the target mycotoxins from different food and feed matrices.

A method for the analysis of mycotoxins in dried fruits, such as plums, raisins, apricots, figs and dates was developed using a modified QuEChERS procedure with LC–MS/MS analysis. Thirteen different mycotoxins were investigated in the fruit samples. The method developed involves homogenizing 5 g of sample with7.5 ml of water containing 1% acetic acid for 3 min. And the mixture obtained was then extracted with 22.5 ml of acetonitrile for 3 min with a vortex. This was followed by the addition of 7.5 g of $MgSO_4$ and 3 g of NaCl and the mixture was shaken manually for 1 hr. The mixture was centrifuged for 10 min at 5000 rpm and the supernatant was collected and evaporated to dryness and was then redissolved with 1 ml of 5 mM aqueous ammonium formate/methanol solution acidified with 1% acetic acid. The resulting solution was filtered through 0.22 μm PTFE filter prior to LC/MS/MS analysis. The limit of detection (LOD) was found to be 0.08–15 μg/kg, limits of quantification (LOQ) was between 0.2–45 μg/kg and recovery in the spiked sample ranged from 60 to 135% with RSD $\leq$ 20 except in beauvericin. Thus, values were below an acceptable limit set by the European Union for the legislated mycotoxins [24].

The occurrence of 16 mycotoxins belonging to different chemical classes was assessed in several nut products using QuEChERS followed by LC–MS/MS analysis. The use of different clean-up sorbents was extensively evaluated. The samples (50 g) were grinded and an aliquot of 1 g of the homogenized sample was transferred into 60 ml centrifuge tube, followed by addition of 5 ml of water and 50 μl of internal standard. Exactly 5 ml of acetonitrile containing 5% formic acid, 2 g of $MgSO_4$ and 0.5 g of NaCl were added and then shaken vigorously by hand for 2 min and centrifuged for 5 min at 3750 rpm. The supernatant (1 ml) was then transferred to the dSPE clean-up tube containing 50 mg of C18 and 50 mg of Z-sep + and centrifuged for 3 min at 1750 rpm. The upper layer was evaporated to dryness under a gentle stream of nitrogen and the dry extract was reconstituted in 250 μl of mixture of methanol/water/acetic acid (97:2:1, v/v) containing 5 mM of ammonium acetate. The method validated using an internal standard calibration method gave linearity between 1.25–500 μg/kg and the detection limits achieved between 0.4–3.5 μg/kg and LOQ ranged from 1.25 to 5 μg/kg for the targeted analytes. The average recoveries ranged between 70 to 93% with RSD $\leq$ 13%. Eleven out of the 16 mycotoxins were found in 37 nut samples, with highest contamination found in cashew sample containing 336.5 μg/kg of deoxynivalenol (DON) [25].

Aflatoxins B1, B2, G1 and G2 and carbamate pesticide contamination were evaluated in 44 samples of bee honey locally produced in Egypt and 9 other countries using QuEChERS followed by HPLC with fluorescence and UV-diode array detector (DAD). Approximately 500 g of each sample was comminuted and 10 g of each was transferred into 50 ml polyethylene tube, followed by addition of 15 ml of acetonitrile and 5 ml of deionized water. The mixture was shaken using a vortex and 6 g of anhydrous magnesium sulphate and 1.5 g of sodium chloride were added and shaken vigorously for 5 min, then centrifuged at 4000 rpm for 4 min. A 4 ml aliquot of the supernatant was transferred to 15 ml centrifuge tube containing 100 mg of PSA and 600 mg of anhydrous magnesium sulphate. The mixture was again vortexed for 3 min and centrifuged for 10 min at 4000 rpm. The supernatant containing the target analytes was derivatized by addition of 50 μl of TFA and 200 μl of hexane, vortexed for 5 min and 1.95 ml of acetonitrile/water (1:9) was added and then centrifuged for 3 min at 4000 rpm. The supernatant was then subjected to HPLC analysis with C18 column and water/methanol/acetonitrile (65/23/12) used a mobile phase at flow rate of 1 ml/min. The recovery results of total aflatoxins and carbamate pesticides were found to range from 88.25 to 92.9% and 78.49 to 98.11%, respectively. The results indicated that all samples were free from any detectable aflatoxin (B1, B2, G1 and G2). On the other hand, promocarb, pirimicarb and aldicarb residues were found in few bee honey samples. All contaminated bee honey samples with carbamate pesticides were under maximum residue limit (MRLs) [26].

A reliable and easy method was developed for the determination of aflatoxins B1 and G1 in maize samples. The mycotoxins content of maize was extracted using QuEChERS coupled to HPLC-FLD with photochemical derivatization. The method used involved weighing 10 g of maize sample into a centrifuge tube and shaking vigorously for 1 min, followed by addition of 1.67 g of sodium acetate and then shaking again for 2 min, the 10 ml 1% acetic in MeCN and 5 ml H_2O of water were added. About 4 g of $MgSO_4$ was added and the mixture was centrifuged for 20 min at 3000*g*. The upper layer was then submitted for HPLC analysis without the clean-up step. The method validation gave linearity between 0.4–20 μg/kg with correlation coefficient greater than 0.99. The limit of detection and quantification were estimated to be 0.08–0.16 and 0.4 μg/kg, respectively, while the average recovery ranged from 79.5–99.73% with RSD ranging from 1.10 to 2.27%. It was discovered that when acetic acid was used with acetonitrile for partitioning, further clean-up is not required, which saves analysis time [27].

Aflatoxins M1, M2, B1, B2, G1, G2 and ochratoxin A were determined in UHT and powdered milk using the modified QuEChERS method coupled to ultra-high performance liquid chromatography–tandem mass spectrometry. For powdered milk, 1.5 g of the sample was transferred into a 50 ml centrifuge tube, followed by addition of 15 ml of deionized water, and the tube was shaken for 30 s. Then, 10 ml of hexane and 15 ml of acetonitrile containing 1% acetic acid were added, followed by 6 g of magnesium sulphate and 1.5 g of sodium chloride and the tube was vigorously shaken for 1 min and then centrifuged for 7 min at 3000 rpm. After centrifugation, the upper layer of hexane was removed and an aliquot of 5 ml of acetonitrile layer was concentrated to dryness with an evaporator at 50°C under gentle flow of nitrogen. The residue was dissolved with 1 ml of mixture of methanol and water (1:1), and the solution was filtered through 0.22 μm polyethylene filter. The filtrate was then subjected to UHPLC procedure using a solution of 5 mM of ammonium formate and

1% acetic acid (phase A) and methanol (phase B) as the mobile phase at a flow rate of 0.3 ml/min. The method yielded good linearity which ranged from 0.1 to 1.5 ng/ml with r^2 greater than 0.99. The LOQ ranged from 0.005 to 0.44 μg/kg, while the LOD ranged from 0.017 to 1.45 μg/kg. The average recoveries for the two types of milk sample range from 72.8 to 121% with RSD = 0.7–16.7%. The analysis of real sample showed the absence of ochratoxin A, aflatoxins B1, B2, G2 and G2 in the milk samples, while aflatoxins M1 were found at concentration levels ranging from 0.005 to 0.0043 and 0.08 to 1.19 μg/kg in UHT and powdered milk, respectively. The aflatoxins found in the milk sample were below the maximum permitted level according to Brazilian legislation, but high according to the EC regulation [28].

The application of QuEChERS sample preparation was optimized and validated for the analysis of mycotoxins in brown rice. The brown rice was blended to a powder sieved and homogenized. An aliquot of 1 g of the homogenized powder sample was transferred into a 50 ml centrifuge tube and 5 ml of water was added and mixed. A 5 ml solution of acetonitrile containing 10% acetic acid was then added to the mixture and vortexed for 1 min at high speed. After the vortexing, 2.0 g anhydrous $MgSO_4$, 0.50 g NaCl, 0.50 g sodium citrate tribasic dihydrate and 0.25 g sodium citrate dibasic sesquihydrate were added and the mixture was vigorously shaken for 1 min, and then centrifuged for 5 min at 1911 × *g*. The supernatant (2 ml) was then transferred into a 15 ml centrifuge tube containing 300 mg anhydrous $MgSO_4$, 50 mg C18, 25 mg of PSA and 25 mg silica. This portion was shaken and centrifuged, and then 1 ml of the supernatant was evaporated to dryness under a stream of nitrogen gas. An aliquot was reconstituted in 1 ml of water with a 1:1 (v/v) ratio of 0.1% (v/v) FA:MeOH and 0.5 μg/l of an SMX IS. The extracted solutions were filtered through 0.22-μm PTFE syringe filters prior to UHPLC–MS–MS analysis. The analytical limits obtained from the method using internal standard calibration method gave linearity in the range of 5–1000 μg/kg, with limit of detection and limit of quantitation ranging from 1.4 to 25 μg/kg and 4.1–55 μg/l, respectively and recoveries in the range of 81–101% with relative standard deviations of 5–19%. Six out of 14 real samples of brown rice were found to be contaminated with at least one of these mycotoxins, ranging from 2.49–5.41 μg/kg of FB1, 4.33 ± 0.04 μg/kg of FB2 and 6.10–14.88 μg/kg of ZON [29].

Aflatoxins were determined in wheat and wheat by-products using in-house validation methods. Three different methods were compared in the study; method 1 involved extraction with chloroform and removal of interfering chemicals by filtration, liquid–liquid partition with hexanemethanol–water and methanol–water-chloroform, and pre-column derivatization with trifluoroacetic acid [30], Method 2 involved extraction with methanol and KCl, purification by filtration with $(NH)_4SO_4$ and Celite, liquid–liquid partition with methanol–water-hexane and methanol–water-chloroform with precolumn derivatization with trifluoroacetic acid; and method 3 involved extraction with methanol:water:acetonitrile (51:40:9, v/v/v) $MgSO_4$ and NaCl, followed by centrifugation and filtration, and the quantification was carried out by HPLC-FLD, without derivatization [31]. Method 3 involved weighing of 2.0 g of thoroughly homogenized sample into a 15 ml polypropylene centrifuge tube followed by addition of 10 ml of extraction solution containing a mixture of methanol:water: acetonitrile (51:40:9, v/v/v) and manually stirred for 1 min. Subsequently, 1.5 g of anhydrous $MgSO_4$ and 0.5 g of NaCl were added and then shaken manually for 1 min. Afterwards, the tube was centrifuged for 5 min, at 4000 rpm, and 1 ml of the extract was collected, filtered through a 0.45 μm membrane and injected into the HPLC-FLD system, without any derivatization procedure. The quantification of the aflatoxins was carried out in an HPLC system, using a fluorescence detector with C18 column isocratic mobile phase, consisting of water: methanol: acetonitrile, at a flow rate of 1.0 ml/min. The methods were validated accruing to the European Commission method EC/401/2006 [32]. The average recoveries were found to be highest in method 1, followed by method 2 and the least was found in method 3, which was observed to be due to lack of derivatization. The method showed a relative standard deviation (RSD) lower than 15% and recovery values in the 70–110% range, with linearity between 1.2 and 24 μg/kg, while the limits of detection and quantification (0.6 and 1.2 μg/kg, respectively) were below the maximum level of aflatoxins allowed in wheat and wheat by-products by the European Commission (4.0 μg/kg) and by the Brazilian legislation (5.0 μg/kg). Using the validated method, aflatoxins were quantified in 20 commercial samples of wheat grains, wheat bran, whole wheat flour and refined wheat flour intended for direct human consumption. Six samples (30%) were positive for aflatoxins and all samples presented levels below the maximum limit stipulated by the Brazilian legislation [33].

QuEChERS LC–MS/MS method was applied for the screening of 12 mycotoxins in cereal products and spices. The samples were homogenized at ambient temperature and 5 g of homogenized samples were separately weighed into a falcon tube and fortified with the working standard solution and left for 10 min. After 10 min, 10 ml of double distilled water and 10 ml of acetonitrile containing 20% acetic acid were added. The mixture was vortexed for 15 min and left for 15 min at −20°C. This was followed by addition of 4 g of $MgSO_4$, 1 g of NaCl and 1 g of sodium citrate tribasic dehydrate and the mixture was shaken for another 1 min and then centrifuged for 10 min at 5000 rpm. The supernatant was transferred into a tube containing 900 mg $MgSO_4$, and 150 mg Supelclean PSA. The mixture was hand shaken and subsequently centrifuged for 5 min at 5000 rpm. An aliquot of 3 ml of the supernatant was evaporated and redissolved in 600 μl of methanol/water (50/50 v/v). The final solution was subjected to HPLC analysis with mobile phase consisting of water (A) and methanol (B). The average recovery of the developed method ranged from 60 to 120% with RSD between 0.026 and 36.7%. The method was found to satisfy the requirements of Commission Regulation (EC) No. 401/2006 and (EC) no. 1881/2006. The screening target concentration (STC) was under maximum permitted levels (MLs) for all mycotoxins validated. All samples were compliant and followed (EC) no. 1881/2006. One sample of maize resulted in OTA at 2.53 μg/Kg, and one sample of black pepper resulted in 1.85 μg/Kg of OTA and the contemporary presence of 0.358 μg/Kg of AFB2 [34].

A reliable and rapid method has been developed for the determination of aflatoxin B1 (AFB1) in four kinds of feedstuffs comprising broken rice, peanuts, corn, and fishmeal. Sample preparation was carried out based on the QuEChERS method with the exclusion of the clean-up step. In this study, AFB1 was extracted using acetonitrile/methanol (40/60 v/v), followed by partitioning with sodium chloride and magnesium sulfate by measuring 10 g of well-milled and homogenized sample into extraction tube followed by addition of 20 ml of acetonitrile/methanol (40/60, v/v%) and the mixture was centrifuged for 3 min at 3000 rpm. Thereafter, 1 g of NaCl and 4 g of anhydrous magnesium sulphate were added and the mixture was shaken and centrifuged again at 3000 rpm for 3 min. The supernatant (1 ml) was evaporated until dry under nitrogen gas. Following that, the precolumn derivatization of AFB1 was carried out and the residue was reconstituted in 900 μl of 10% acetonitrile followed by addition of 100 μl of trifluoroacetic acid and then incubated for 15 min at 15°C. The derivatized solution was then centrifuged at 1000*g* for 5 min before HPLC-FLD analysis. The method validated yielded recovery of all feedstuffs achieved a range of 82.50–109.85% with relative standard deviation ranging from 0.57–11% for all analytes at a concentration of 20−100 ng/g. The limit of detection (LOD) ranged from 0.2 to 1.2 ng/g and limit of quantitation (LOQ) ranged from 0.3 to 1.5 ng/g. The validated method was successfully applied to a total of 120 samples. The occurrence of AFB1 contamination was found at the following concentrations: in broken rice (0.44−2.33 ng/g), peanut (3.97−106.26 ng/g), corn (0.88−50.29 ng/g), and fishmeal (1.06−10.35 ng/g). It was suggested as an alternative to expensive and time-consuming methods by using immune affinity columns or two steps of liquid/solid extraction procedure [35].

A rapid method is proposed for determining aflatoxins B1 and M1 in milk and dairy products by HPLC with fluorimetric detection. A sample of about 5.0 g was collected into a 50 ml test tube and 5 ml of water and 10 ml of acetonitrile were added; the tube was sealed and shaken for 30 min. Then a mixture of salts consisting of 1.0 g of NaCl, 1.0 g of trisodium citrate dihydrate and 0.5 g of disodium hydrogen citrate sesquihydrate was added. The test tube was shaken for 1 min and centrifuged for 45 min at 5000 rpm. An 8.0 ml portion of an extract from the upper layer was collected and taken into a 15 ml centrifuge tube, already charged with a mixture of 950 mg of $MgSO_4$, 200 mg of adsorbent Bondesil PSA, and adsorbent C18 (200 mg, for raw milk or dairy products or 400 mg for cheese). The tube was shaken vigorously for 30 s and centrifuged for 5 min at 2700 rpm. Then 3.0 ml of an acetonitrile extract and 500 μl of chloroform were put into a 15 ml centrifuge tube charged with 7.0 ml of deionized water using a syringe. The mixture was shaken for 20−30 s, kept in an ultrasonic bath for 2 min, and centrifuged for 10 min at 2700 rpm; the bottom layer was collected into a microvial and evaporated to dryness in a flow of nitrogen; the residue was dissolved in 50 μl of acetonitrile and subjected to chromatography analysis. The method gave average recoveries ranging from 51.2–75.7%. The limit of detection and quantitation were estimated to range from 0.01−0.1 and 0.03–0.3 μg/kg, with linearity ranging from 0.03 to 10 μg/kg and a correlation coefficient greater than 0.998. Aflatoxin B1 was found in samples of cheese only, and M1 was found in all the samples studied. The concentration of aflatoxins did not exceed the maximum permissible concentration legalized in Russia [36].

A suitable method for routine analysis of aflatoxins M1, M2, B1, B2, G1 and G2 in peanut by ultra-high performance liquid chromatography–tandem mass spectrometry was developed and validated. The sample preparation was performed using a triple partitioning (water/acetonitrile/hexane) modified Quick Easy Cheap Effective Rugged and Safe (QuEChERS) method. For the first time, this method is reportedly used for aflatoxins analysis in peanuts. To 5 g of the sample, weighed in a 50 ml centrifuge tube, were added 10 ml of ultrapure water, 10 ml of hexane and 15 ml of acetonitrile; the tube was then shaken for 30 s; a mixture of 4 g of magnesium sulphate and 1.5 g of sodium chloride was added, the tube was immediately shaken vigorously using a vortex for1 min and then centrifuged at 3000 rpm for 7 min. An aliquot of 5 ml of the acetonitrile phase was evaporated to dryness under a gentle flow of nitrogen at 45°C and then the residue was dissolved with 2 ml of methanol/water (1:1, v/v). The solution thus obtained was filtered through a 0.22 μm polyethylene filter before injection to HPLC. Satisfactory recoveries ranged from 71.3 to 101.3%, with a relative standard deviation ranging from 1.5–12.4% obtained for the target aflatoxins. The determination coefficients were ≥ 0.99 which showed good linearity (0.15–15 μg/l). The LOD and LOQ varied from 0.03 to 0.26 ng/g and 0.1 to 0.88 ng/g, respectively [37].

Two multi-residue methods were developed and compared for the analysis of 17 mycotoxins in cereals by liquid chromatography-electrospray ionization tandem mass spectrometry. The extraction procedures considered were a QuEChERS-like method and one using accelerated solvent extraction (ASE). The QuEChERS-like extraction procedure involved weighing 5 g of the sample into a 50 ml tube followed by addition of 10 ml of water and 10 ml of acetonitrile containing 0.5% acetic acid. The mixture was vigorously shaken and 5 g of $MgSo_4$/NaCl (4:1, w/w) was added and shaken again, followed by centrifugation at 4000 rpm for 15 min. For clean-up, 5 ml of the supernatant was transferred into a 15 ml tube and was defatted with 5 ml of n-hexane under agitation and then centrifuged for 1 min at 4000 rpm. Subsequently, 1 ml of the supernatant (equivalent to 0.5 g of sample) was transferred into a tube and evaporated to dryness at 40°C under stream of nitrogen and the residue was reconstituted with 75 μl of methanol, sonicated for a few min and 75 μl of water was added. The whole extract was then transferred into a 1.5 ml tube and centrifuged at 8500 rpm for 10 min. The resulting supernatant (60 μl) was then further diluted with water (140 μl) and recentrifuged (8500 rpm 10 min), and the clear supernatant was transferred into an HPLC amber glass vial for further LC-ESI-MS/MS analysis. The method validation estimated using the optimized method gave recovery ranging from 73 to 130% with RSD of 0 to 18%. The LOQ was between 0.5–100 μg/kg. The two-extraction procedure was found to give similar performances in terms of linearity ($r^2 > 0.98$), both methods showed high extraction efficiency in a broad range of cereal-based products and with comparable sensitivity. Nevertheless, the easiness-to-handle of these extraction methods was definitely in favor of the QuEChERS-like procedure, since it requires less reagents and glassware and involves less intermediate steps. Consequently, a higher sample throughput was possible, with up to 40 individual samples extracted over one working day as compared to the 24 individual samples processed over one and a half working days by the ASE procedure. On a routine basis, the QuEChERS-like method constitutes undeniably the best option [38].

The presence of mycotoxin and pesticide residues was analyzed in milk using QuEChERS method. The efficiency was evaluated using the original QuEChERS and acetate buffered methods. For the original method, 10 ml of milk was extracted with 10 ml of acetonitrile, stirred for 1 min, followed by addition of 1 g of NaCl and 4 g of $MgSO_4$, with stirring at vortex for 1 min and centrifuged at 5000 rpm for 5 min. And for the acetate buffered QuEChERS method, 15 ml of milk was extracted with 15 ml of acetonitrile containing 1% acetic acid, the mixture was stirred for 1 min, followed by addition of 6 g of $MgSO_4$ and 1.5 g of sodium acetate with stirring at vortex for 1 min and centrifuged at 5000 rpm for 5 min. After centrifugation, 2 ml of the supernatant was transferred to a centrifuge tube containing 150 mg of $MgSO_4$, 50 mg of PSA and 50 mg of C18. The mixture was stirred for 30 s and centrifuged at 5000 rpm for 5 min. The extract was filtered through a PTFE membrane, and then 1 ml of extract was transferred to a vial, evaporated to dryness and redissolved in 1 ml of mixture of acetonitrile/ammonium formate +0.01 formic acid (95/5 v/v) and subjected to UPLC. The original QuEChERS method was found to be more efficient than the acetate buffered and was adopted for method validation. The developed method was validated according to the analytical quality assurance manual of the Brazilian Ministry of Agriculture and the European Commission Decision No 2002/657/EC. The average recovery values were found between 85 and 97% for aflatoxin M1, with RSD ranging from 14.5 to 16.3%. The limit of detection and quantification were 0.02 and 0.04, with linearity ranging from 0 to 1.0 μg/kg and correlation coefficient of 0.997. Residues of aflatoxin M1 were also found in field samples at levels below the established maximum residue limit [39].

A simultaneous analysis method was developed for faster and cheaper determination of 13 different mycotoxins in feedstuffs using QuEChERS followed by LC–MS/MS. For sample preparation, 5 g of the freeze-dried samples were accurately weighed and transferred into 50 ml tube followed by addition of 10 ml of water containing 10% formic acid, and 10 ml of acetonitrile. The mixture was shaken for 30 min, and different combinations of salts were then added (salt 1 containing 4 g anhydrous magnesium sulfate and 1 g sodium chloride; salt 2, 4 g anhydrous magnesium sulfate, 1 g sodium chloride, 1 g trisodium citrate dihydrate and 0.5 g disodium hydrogen citrate sesquihydrate; salt 3, 6 g anhydrous magnesium sulfate and 1.5 g sodium acetate). The mixture was shaken for 1 min and then centrifuged at 4000 rpm for 10 min. For the cleanup, 1 ml of the supernatant was transferred into a tube containing 25 mg of PSA and 25 mg of C18 and then centrifuged for 5 min at 10,000 rpm. A 400 μl aliquot of the supernatant was then transferred to a microtube and mixed with 500 μl of distilled water and 100 μl of acetonitrile. The solution was then filtered through 0.20 μl PTFE syringe filter and was then subjected to LC–MS/MS analysis. The salt containing magnesium sulfate and sodium chloride (salt 1) was found to be the most efficient and was used for method validation. The analytical method was validated following SANTE/11813/2017 and CODEX guidelines. Average recovery was found between 70.1 and 115.6% with RSD –0.1–11.3, the LOD ranged from 0.8333 to 16.7 μg/l, the LOQ ranged from 2.5 to 50 μg/l, while linearity ranged from 0.5 to 500 μg/l with r^2 greater than 0.99. Mycotoxins were found in the 39 samples but did not exceed the maximum residual level (MRL) criterion set by Korean Food and Drug Administration [40].

A simple and efficient method for determining multiple mycotoxins was developed using a QuEChERS-based procedure for the analysis of mycotoxins in vegetable oil using high-performance liquid chromatography–tandem mass spectrometry. Different extraction procedures were studied and optimized by spiking 16 analytes into blank matrix. A 1 g sample was weighed into a 30 ml centrifuge tube and then spiked with a mycotoxin's standard mixture at different concentrations and was left for 1 h for equilibration. Then 2 ml of water was added vortexed for 1 min and 8 ml of acetonitrile was thereafter added and the extraction was achieved using end-over-end shaker for 20 min. Subsequently, 4 g of anhydrous Na_2SO_4 and 1 g of NaCl were added. The tube was capped immediately, vortexed for 2 min and then centrifuged at 5000 rpm for 5 min. The supernatant (8 ml) was transferred into a 15 ml centrifuge tube containing different sorbents (C18, PSA and neutral Al_2O_3, containing 100, 150 and 200 mg, respectively) and the tube was shaken by hand for 5 min and centrifuged for 5 min at 8000 rpm and 4 ml of the extract (upper layer) was transferred into a glass tube and evaporated to dryness under a stream of N_2 and then reconstituted by addition of 1 ml of mixture of acetonitrile/water (1:1, v/v%). The most efficient extraction was achieved with 85% of acetonitrile solution and C18 as cleanup sorbent, which allowed average recovery between 72.8–105.8% with RSD less than 7% (RSD = 0.2–6.3). The limit of detection (LOD) ranged from 0.04 to 2.9 ng/g, while limit of quantitation ranged from 0.12 to 10 ng/g, with linearity ranging from 0.2 to 500 ng/g and r^2 greater than 0.99. Zearalenone (ZEN), aflatoxin B1 (AFB1), aflatoxin B2 (AFB2), aflatoxin G1(AFG1) and α-zearalenol (α-ZOL) were detected, with maximum concentrations of 0.59 (AFG1)– 42.5 (ZEN) ng/g. The method developed has the advantages of high sensitivity, accuracy and selectivity, and it can be applied to the target screening of mycotoxins in real samples [41].

A new method for the determination and analysis of ochratoxin A (OTA) in cereals and cereal products, based on the use of the QuEChERS procedure enhanced with HPLC-FLD was developed. Cereal samples were prepared similar to the previous published aflatoxin QuEChERS method with some modifications. The modified QuEChERS involves three steps; First step includes measuring a thoroughly homogenized cereal sample (1 g) weighed in a polypropylene centrifuge tube (15 ml). Subsequently, they were extracted via the following steps (II to IV). Step II: 3.0 ml of 20:70:10 (%, v/v) water/acetonitrile/acetic acid mixture was added, and the centrifuge tube was shaken for 1 min to ensure that the solvent has mixed thoroughly with the entire sample, for complete extraction of the analyte. Step III: 0.8 g of anhydrous MgSO4 and 0.2 g of NaCl were added to the mixture and the shaking procedure was repeated for 1 min to facilitate the extraction and partitioning of the ochratoxin A into the organic layer. Step IV: The extract was centrifuged for 5 min at 4000 rpm and 0.5 ml of the upper organic layer was filtered through a 0.45 μm nylon syringe filter prior to HPLC analysis. The linearity of the developed method ranged from 3.75 to 120 μg/l with r^2 greater than 0.99. The recoveries obtained ranged from 85.2 ± 1.2 to 109.8 ± 2.9%, with a relative standard deviation (RSD) of less than 12%. The LOQ were from 0.60 to 2.08 μg/kg, with LOD ranging from 0.18 to 0.62 μg/kg [42].

A combination of modified QuEChERS with ultrahigh-performance liquid chromatography–tandem mass spectrometry (UPLC–MS/MS) has been used for simultaneous detection of 20 mycotoxins in grains. A series of different types of magnetic (Fe_3O_4) nanoparticles modified with multiwalled carbon nanotubes (Fe_3O_4-MWCNTs) were designed as modified QuEChERS adsorbents for facile and efficient purification and for target interferences removal in the matrices. A 5.0 g of grains was added into 50 ml centrifugation tubes. Acetonitrile/water (25 ml; 80:20, v/v, 1% acetic acid) was added, and the tube was vigorously shaken with a vortex mixer for 1 min. Then, after citrate buffer containing 4 g of MgSO4, 1 g of NaCl, 1 g of $Na_3Cit{\cdot}2H_2O$, and 0.5 g of $Na_2Cit{\cdot}1.5H_2O$ were added, the mixture was shaken vigorously for 1 min followed by centrifugation at 8000 rpm for 5 min. Fe_3O_4-MWCNTs (20 mg) and 1.0 ml of the purified supernatant were added to a 2.0 ml microcentrifuge. The mixture was mixed vigorously for 1 min and separated by a magnetic force created by a magnet. The solution was passed through a 0.22 μm PTFE membrane filter, and 5 μl of the final solution was analyzed by UPLC -MS/MS. The method validated in accordance with the Commission regulation 401/2006/EC and SANCO guidelines 12,571/2013 gave linear range of 0.1–500 ng/g with r^2 greater than 0.99. The method yielded good recovery between 73.5 and 112.9% and RSD ranging from 1.3 to 12.7%, with the LODs and LOQs for the 20 mycotoxins ranging from 0.0006 to 1.6337 and from 0.0021 to 5.4457 ng/g, respectively. The developed method was compared with published works, where other adsorbent materials and the developed method were found to have a wider linear range and lower LOQ [43].

Five mycotoxins were detected in different food matrices obtained from Malaysian market using validated QuEChERS-LC–MS/MS. Low-fat samples were prepared by measuring 2 g of homogeneous solid food (or 2 ml liquid sample) were weighed and transferred to a 50 ml centrifuge tube. Then, 10 ml of acetonitrile acidified with 1% acetic acid and 7.5 ml of cold water were added to the tube, shaken for 1 min, and vortexed for 4 min, followed by the addition of 4 g of anhydrous $MgSO_4$ and 1 g of sodium chloride and shaken for 3 min. The mixture was then centrifuged for 6 min at 7500 rpm. Exactly 4 ml of the supernatant was pipetted out and added to a 15 ml centrifuge tube containing 0.2 g PSA and 0.6g of fine powder anhydrous $MgSO_4$. The extract was further shaken for 2 min and centrifuged at 4000 rpm for 5 min. Then, 2.5 ml of the supernatant was evaporated to dryness by a rotary evaporator and reconstituted with 1 ml of methanol and filtered through a 0.22 μm nylon syringe filter prior to the LC–MS/MS analysis. For samples with high-fat content, 2.5 g of the homogenized samples was weighed and transferred to a 50 ml polypropylene centrifuge tube. Then, 20 ml aqueous acetonitrile (containing 1% acetic acid) solution (80:20, v/v) was added to the mixture and shaken for 30 min at 300 rpm. The mixture was then centrifuged for 5 min at 8000 rpm and the supernatant was transferred into a clean vial. The extraction process was repeated twice. Then, 4 g of magnesium sulfate, 1 g of sodium chloride, 1 g of sodium citrate, and 0.5 g of sodium hydrogen citrate sesquihydrate were added to the combined supernatant and shaken for 1 min. The fat content was removed by treating the extracts with 20 ml of hexane (2 times), vortexing for 1 min and followed by standing for 5 min to separate the hexane from the extract. For the dispersive SPE clean-up, the bottom layer was transferred into a clean tube that contained 150 mg of C18 sorbent and 900 mg of magnesium sulfate. The cloudy solution was shaken for 1 min and centrifuged at 8000 rpm for 5 min. The supernatant was transferred into a clean tube and washed twice with 5 ml of acetonitrile. The mixture was evaporated to dryness by a rotary evaporator and reconstituted with 1 ml of methanol and filtered through a 0.22 μm nylon syringe filter prior to LC–MS/MS analysis. The method demonstrated good sensitivity of concentration range ranging from 1 to 30 μg/kg ($r^2 > 0.996$), with LOD that ranged from 0.05 to 0.1 μg/kg, and LOQ that ranged from 0.08 to 0.3 μg/kg, which was found to be lower than the allowable maximum limit for aflatoxin. The recovery of the target analytes ranges from 81.94 to 101.67%, intra-day and inter-day precision range from 0.12 to 7.25% and 0.23 to 10.28%, respectively. The developed method was compared to other QuEChERS methods, and the developed method revealed excellent overall results. Aflatoxins were detected in raisin, pistachio, peanut, wheat flour, spice, and chili samples with concentrations ranging from 0.45 to 16.93 μg/kg. Trace concentration of ochratoxin A was found in wheat flour and peanut samples which ranged from 1.2 to 3.53 μg/kg. Some of the tested food samples contained mycotoxins above the European legal maximum limit [44].

A method was developed to simultaneously quantify different mycotoxins in 30 and 10 corn flour samples using modified QuEChERS in combination with an LC–MS/MS technique. About 5 g of homogenized corn flour sample was placed into the falcon tube (50 ml). The appropriate concentrations of the mixed working standard solution (for spiking) and aflatoxin M1 (internal standard) were added to the falcon tube. After an hour, 15 ml of acetonitrile (79%):water (20%):formic acid (1%) (v/v/v) were added, this was followed by addition of 1 g of sodium chloride. The obtained mixture was shaken vigorously for 10 min at 340 rpm. Then, 5 g of magnesium sulfate was added to the mixture. Subsequently, the sample was vortexed for 2 min and centrifuged for 10 min at 1585*g* at 5°C. An aliquot of 5 ml of the extract was transferred to a Falcon (15 ml) tube containing 1 g $MgSO_4$ and 0.3 g PSA Again, the samples were vortexed and centrifuged as described previously. Afterwards, 4 ml of the extract was poured into a vial and then evaporated to dryness using nitrogen gas. Afterwards, reconstitution of the residue using methanol (1 ml) was carried out. Then, 20 μl of solution was injected into the LC–MS/MS after filtering through 0.2 μm syringe filter. The method validated using SANTE/11945/2015 document gave linearity between 2 and 1800 ng/g with r^2 greater than 0.99. The LOQ and LOD were respectively found 2–75 ng/g and 0.6—25 ng/g. The recoveries were in the range 92.9–103.8% and RSD 3.7–20%. AFB1, OTA, and ZEA were detected and quantified in 23 (76.6%), 6 (20%), and 14 (46%) of 30 samples, with average contamination of 154.1, 25, and 358.7 ng/g, respectively. The co-occurrence of AFB1 + ZEA and AFB1 + OTA + ZEA was noted in 20% and 23% of corn samples, respectively. The measured level of contamination for DON and T-2 toxin in corn flour samples did not exceed the maximum tolerated level [45].

A fast, easy, and cheap method for the simultaneous determination and quantification of aflatoxins in cereal-derived products was developed by Annumziata and co-workers using QuEChERS extraction coupled with LC–MS/MS. The sample was prepared by measuring 2 g of the homogenized sample into a 50 ml tube and was spied with the internal standard. The fortified sample was kept in the dark for 15 min, to allow equilibration of IS with the matrix. Then 10 ml of water containing 0.1% formic acid was added and shaked the mixture for 3 min. Then 10 ml of acetonitrile were added, and the sample was further shaken for 3 min. This was followed by addition of 4 g MgSO4 and 1 g NaCl and the mixture was immediately shaken for 2 min to prevent agglomerates from forming during MgSO4 hydration and then centrifuged at 3500 × *g* for 10 min. About 2 ml of the extract was evaporated under a stream of nitrogen and the residue was constituted by addition of 200 μl of a solution of methanol/water containing 5 mM ammonium formate and 0.1% formic acid (10:90, v/v) and was then filtered through a 0.45-μm polyvinylidene fluoride filter into a vial. The developed method was validated using regulation EC 888/2004, and it yield average recoveries ranging from 83.8 to 102.9% with RSD between 14.3 and 15.7%. The LOD and LOQ were 0.5–100 and 1–200 μg/kg, respectively, and linearity ranging from 0 to 140 μg/kg with r^2 greater than 0.99. The method was then applied for the analysis of 21 cereal-derived products purchased on the Italian market, which were correctly packaged and labeled as intended for human consumption. The co-occurrence of more than one mycotoxin in the analyzed samples could represent a risk for consumers, and the described method could be a valid alternative for their simultaneous detection in the framework of official control [46].

The possibility of applying QuEChERS extraction of 2 mycotoxins in cereals and subsequent detection using enzyme-linked immunosorbent assay (ELISA) has been investigated. Each homogenized cereal sample was accurately weighed (4.0 g, precision: 0.01 mg) into 50 ml centrifuge tubes, followed by addition of 16 ml of mixture of acetonitrile/methanol (80:20 v/v) and the mixture was shaken for by vortex for 1 min. Then QuEChERS extraction kit (6 g of magnesium sulphate, 1.5 g of sodium chloride, 1.5 g of sodium citrate dihydrate and 1 g of sodium citrate sesquihydrate) was added and the tube was shaken vigorously for 5 min and then centrifuged at 8000 rpm for 10 min. An aliquot of 8 ml of the supernatant was transferred into 15 ml centrifuge tube containing 300 mg PSA and 100 mg $MgSO_4$ anhydrous and the tube was vortexed vigorously for 1 min. Subsequently, the sample was centrifuged at 8000 rpm for 3 min. And then, 4 ml of the upper organic solvent layer was transferred to a vial, evaporated to near dryness under a gentle stream of N_2 and reconstituted with 1 ml of MeOH: PBS (10:90, v/v) for ELISA analysis. The recovery of the method ranged from 83.55 to 106.93% with RSD between 1.11 and 7.42%. The sensitive and specific ELISA was applied to the determination of ZEN and DON in cereal. For ZEN, the linear range was 13.64–104.48 ng/ml, the LOD was 2.58 ng/ml, and for DON, the linear range was 35.65–983.52 ng/ml, the LOD was 17.31 ng/ml. The ELISA method for determination of ZEN and DON was compared with a standard HPLC method. The values obtained from the two detection systems for ZEN and DON entirely fit an excellent linear relationship, with a regression equation of $y = 1.0281x - 0.2897$ (correlation coefficient is 0.9955) for ZEN and a regression equation of $y = 0.9952x + 4.4193$ (correlation coefficient is 0.9984) for DON, further confirming the reliability of ELISA [47].

A modified QuEChERS (Quick, Easy, Cheap, Effective, Rugged and Safe) method was developed for the simultaneous determination of veterinary drugs, pesticides and mycotoxins in eggs by ultrahigh-pressure liquid chromatography–tandem mass spectrometry (UPLC–MS/MS). In the purification procedure, magnetic multiwalled carbon nanotubes (Fe_3O_4-MWCNTs) were used as adsorbents, and an external magnet was utilized to achieve a faster adsorbent separation, compared to the traditional centrifugation process. About 5.0 g of the homogenized sample were weighed into a 50 ml centrifuge tube. Subsequently, 5 ml of 0.1 mM Na_2EDTA solution and 20 ml of 1% of HOAc in ACN were added. The mixture was then vortexed for 1 min, followed by addition of 4.0 g of Na_2SO_4 and 1.0 g of NaCl, and the tubes were vortexed immediately for another 1 min. The sample was then centrifuged at 6000 rpm for 10 min, and 2 ml of supernatant was transferred into a 5 ml dispersive tube containing 15 mg of Fe_3O_4-MWCNTs composite. The mixture was vortexed for 1 min, and then the adsorbents were separated quickly from the solution with an external magnet. Finally, 1 ml of the above solution was diluted with 1 ml of aqueous methanol solution (50/50, v/v), and the solution was finally filtered by a 0.22 μm PTFE syringe filter for UPLC–MS/MS analysis. The recoveries of all analytes were in the range of 60.5–114.6%, while the recoveries for the mycotoxins varied from 71.8 to 100.0%, at three fortified levels with relative standard deviations (RSDs) ranging from 1.6 to 17.3%. The LOQs for all the target analytes ranged from 0.1 to 17.3 μg/kg, while it was found between 0.2 and 11.8 for mycotoxins and the linearity ranged from 1 to 100 μg/kg. This method was successfully applied to the analysis of egg samples, demonstrating its applicability and suitability for the routine analysis of multiclass residues in egg samples [48].

A high-throughput method for the simultaneous determination of 26 mycotoxins in sesame butter was developed by coupling the modified QuEChERS method with ultra-high performance liquid chromatography triple quadrupole mass spectrometry (UHPLC–MS/MS). The sample (2.5 g) was weighed into a centrifuge tube and sequentially extracted using two different solutions. The sample was first extracted using 20 ml of a mixture of acetonitrile/water solution (80:20, v/v) containing 0.1% formic acid for 30 min by continuous shaking. The tube was shaken with shaker at 300 rpm, followed by centrifugation at 8000 rpm for 5 min. The supernatant was then transferred to a clean vial. The remaining residue was further extracted using 5 ml of an acetonitrile aqueous solution (20:80, v/v) containing 0.1% formic acid for an additional 30 min with continuous shaking at 300 rpm, followed by centrifugation at 8000 rpm for 5 min. The two supernatants were combined before being subjected to salting out and fat removal. About 4 g of magnesium sulfate, 1 g of sodium chloride, 1 g of sodium citrate and 0.5 g of sodium hydrogen citrate sesquihydrate was added to the supernatant with immediate vortexing for 1 min to enhance the partition of the mycotoxins into the organic layer. The tube was then centrifuged at 8000 rpm for 5 min. The upper layer was collected and mixed with 20 ml of hexane, followed by vortexing for 1 min to remove fat. After standing for 5 min, the upper layer was removed, and the lower layer was transferred into a tube containing 150 mg of C18 and 900 mg of magnesium sulfate for the dSPE clean-up. The cloudy solution was vortexed for 1 min and then centrifuged. The resulting supernatant was decanted into a clean tube. The dispersive tube was washed twice with 5 ml of acetonitrile, sequentially. The washing solution was then collected and combined with the supernatant. The resulting sample solution was subjected to drying at 40°C using the rotary evaporator. Finally, the residue was sequentially dissolved in 1.5 ml of methanol and 1.0 ml of water, and the resultant solution was passed through a 0.22-m nylon filter for further analysis using UHPLC–MS/MS. The calibration curves were prepared in a blank matrix with a series of concentrations between 0.5 and 500 ng/ml with good linear relationships were achieved with linear regression coefficients (r^2) of 0.994 or higher. The LOQs of the samples ranged from 0.11 to 21.74 μg/kg, while the LOD ranged from 0.05 to 7.25 μg/kg. The recovery values (60–111.70%) are within 60–120%, except those of FB2 and PAX at two higher levels and that of ST at the lowest level. All of the RSDs (0–14.6%) were within 15%, with the majority of values (96% of the total) within 10%. The results showed that 10 peanut butter samples were all contaminated with AFs and FBs with total concentrations in the

Aflatoxins	Sample Matrix	QuEChERS procedure	Clean-Up method	Instrumental analysis	Linearity (μg/kg) (R^2)	Recovery (%) (RSD %)	LOD (μg/kg)	LOQ (μg/kg)	Reference
AF(B1, B2, G1, G2)	Cereals, peanuts, peanut butter, nuts, sesame seeds, pistachio nuts, green coffee	1 g sample, 3 ml, ACN/H_2O, (40/60, v/v%), 1.32 g $MgSO_4$, 0.25 g NaCl	Filter through 0.45 μm Nylon syringe filter	HPLC-FLD	0.059–100 (>0.993)	76.3–98.0 (<10)	0.06–0.35	0.18–1.17	[2]
B1, M1	Milk	10 ml sample 4.0 g Na_2SO_4, 1.2 g NaCl, 2.5 ml H_2O, 5.0 ml ACN (3.35% HCOOH)	Supernatant + MeOH: H2O (70:30 v/v) then filtered	HPLC-Q-orbitrap MS	0.002–20 μg/l (>0.999)	75–96 (7–16)	0.001	–0.002	[20]
AF(B1, B2, G1, G2), FFB1 B2), DON, OTA (ZON)	Brown rice	1 g sample, 2.0 g $MgSO_4$, 0.50 g NaCl, 0.50 g sodium citrate tribasic dihydrate and 0.25 g sodium citrate dibasic sesquihydrate 5 ml 10% (v/v) HOAc in ACN	300 mg $MgSO_4$, 50 mg C18, 25 mg PSA and 25 mg silica	UHPLC–MS/MS	5.0–1000 (n.r)	81–101 (5–19)	1.4–2.5	4.1–8.5	[29]
AF(B1, B2, G1, G2)	Rice	3.3 g sample 6.6 ml H_2O, 10 ml ACN, 4 g $MgSO_4$, 1 g NaCl	150 mg PSA. 600 mg $MgSO_4$	HPLC-FLD	4–40 (>0.999)	102–128 (<12)	0.05–6.0	0.15–3.0	[21]
11 mycotoxins	Plant-based beverages	50 ml sample 4 g $MgSO_4$, 1 g NaCl, 10 ml ACN(1% HCOOH)	Supernatant filtered through 0.2 μm nylon filter	UHPLC–MS/MS	0.05–2000 μg/l	80–91 (n.r)	0.02–0.4 μg/l	0.05–15 0 μg/l	[23]
15 mycotoxins		10 g sample, 40 ml 84% ACN/H_2O	Supernatant evaporated and reconstituted with	HPLC–MS/MS	0.5–400 (n.r)	80.1–95.5 (10.5–19.6)	0.70–5.0	n.r	[22]

Aflatoxins	Sample Matrix	QuEChERS procedure	Clean-Up method	Instrumental analysis	Linearity (µg/kg) (R^2)	Recovery (%) (RSD %)	LOD (µg/kg)	LOQ (µg/kg)	Reference
			ethyl acetate and cyclohexane (50:50 v/v) and filtered through 0.45 µm nylon filter						
13 mycotoxins	plums, raisins, apricots, figs and dates	5 g sample, 7.5 ml H_2O, 1% HOAc, 22.5 ml ACN, 7.5 g $MgSO_4$, 3 g NaCl	Supernatant redissolved in 1 ml ammonioum formate/ methanol +1% HOAc, filtered through 0.22 µm filter	LC–MS/MS	n.r (>0.998)	60–135 (≤ 20)	0.08–15	0.2–45	[24]
16 mycotoxins	almonds, peanuts, walnuts, hazelnuts, pecan nuts, cashews, Brazil nut, pine nuts	1 g sample, 5 ml H_2O, 5 ml ACN (5% HCOOH) 2 g $MgSO_4$, 0.5 g NaCl	50 mg C18, 50 mg Z-sep$^+$,	LC-MS/MS	11.25–500 (>0.970)	70–93 (≤13)	0.4–3.5	1.25–5	[25]
AF(B1, B2, G1, G2)	Honeybee	10 g sample, 15 ml ACN, 5 ml H_2O, 6 g $MgSO_4$, 1.5 g NaCl	100 mg PSA, 600 mg $MgSO_4$	HPLC-UV-DAD	n.r	88.25–92.9	n.r	n.r	[26]
AF(B1, G1)	maize	10 g sample, 1.67 g NaOAc, 10 ACN (1% HOAc), 4 g $MgSO_4$	No clean-up	HPLC-FLD	0.4–20 µg/l (>0.99)	79.5–99.73 (1.10–2.27)	0.08–16	n.r	[27]
AF(B1, B2, G1, G2, M1, M2)	Peanut	5 g sample, 10 ml H_2O, 10 ml hexane, 15 ml ACN), 4 g $MgSO_4$, 1,5 g NaCl	Supernatant dried +2 ml MeOH/H_2O and filtered	UHPLC–MS/MS	0.15–15 µg/l (>0.99)	71.3–100.3 (1.5–12.4)	0.03–0.26	0.10–0.88	[37]

Aflatoxins	Sample Matrix	QuEChERS procedure	Clean-Up method	Instrumental analysis	Linearity (µg/kg) (R^2)	Recovery (%) (RSD %)	LOD (µg/kg)	LOQ (µg/kg)	Reference
AF(B1, B2, G1, G2)	Wheat and wheat by-products	2 g sample, 10 ml $MeOH/H_2O/ACN$, 1.5 g $MgSO_4$, 0.5 g NaCl	Filtered through a 0.45 µm	HPLC-FD	1.2–24 (>0.99)	70–110 (>15)	0.6	1.2	[33]
12 mycotoxins	Maize, wheat, black pepper, coffee	5 g sample, 10 ml H_2O, 10 ml ACN, (20% HOAc), 4 g $MgSO_4$, 1 g NaCl, 1 g sodium citrate tribasic dehydrate	900 mg $MgSO_4$, 150 mg PSA	UHPLC–MS/MS	0.8–2000 µg/l (>0.99)	60–120 (0.026–36.7)	n.r	n.r	[34]
AFB1	Rice, peanut, corn, fishmeal	10 g sample, 20 ml ACN/MeOH (40/60%), 4 g $MgSO_4$, 1 g NaCl	No clean up step	HPLC-FLD	5–100 (>0.98)	82.50–109.85 (0.57–11)	0.2–1.2	0.3–1.5	[35]
AF(B1, M1)	Milk, dairy products	5 g sample, 5 ml H_2O, 1 g NaCl, 1 g trisodium citrate dehydrate, 0.5 g disodium hydrogen citrate sesquihydrate	950 mg MgSO4, 200 mg Bondesil PSA, 200–400 mg C18	HPLC-FLD	0.03–10	51.2–75.7 (n.r)	0.01–0.1	0.03–0.3	[36]
AF(B1, B2, G1, G2, M1, M2)	Milk	1.5 g sample, 10 ml H_2O, 10 ml Hexane, 15 ml ACN 1% HOAc), 6 g $MgSO_4$, 1.5 g NaCl	Supernatant dried +5 ml $MeOH/H_2O$, filtered through a 0.22 µm polyethylene filter	UHPLC–MS/MS	1. – 1.5 µg/l (≥ 0.99)	72.8–121 (0.7–16.7)	0.017–1.45	0.005–0.44	[28]
17 mycotoxins	Cereal	5 g sample, 10 ml H_2O, 10 ml ACN (0.5% HOAc), 4 g $MgSO_4$, 1 g NaCl,	Evaporated to dryness and reconstituted with 75 µl methanol	LC–MS/MS	0–10,000 (>0.98)	73–130 (0–18)	n.r	0.5–100	[38]

Aflatoxins	Sample Matrix	QuEChERS procedure	Clean-Up method	Instrumental analysis	Linearity (μg/kg) (R^2)	Recovery (%) (RSD %)	LOD (μg/kg)	LOQ (μg/kg)	Reference
AFM1	Milk	10 ml sample, 10 ml ACN, 1 g NaCl, 4 g $MgSO_4$	150 mg $MgSO_4$, 50 mg PSA, 50 mg C18.	LC–MS/MS	0–1.0	85–97 (14.5–16.3)	0.02	0.4	[39]
13 mycotoxins	Feedstuff	5 g sample, 10 ml H_2O (10% HCOOH, 10 ml ACN, 1 g NaCl, 4 g $MgSO_4$	25 mg PSA, 25 mg C18	LC–MS/MS	0.5–500 μg/l (>0.98)	70.1–115.6 (0.1–11.3	0.8333–16.7 μg/l	2.5–50 μg/l	[40]
16 mycotoxins	Vegetable oil	1 g sample, 2 ml H_2O, 18 ml ACN, 4 g Na_2SO_4, 1 g NaCl	100 mg C18	HPLC-MS	0.2–500 (>0.99)	72.8–105.8 (0.2–6.3)	0.04–2.9	0.12–1-	[41]
OTA	Cereals	1 g sample, 3 ml H_2O/ACN/HOAc, 0.8 g $MgSO_4$, 0.2 g NaCl	Filtered through a 0.45 μm nylon syringe filter	HPLC-FLD	3.75–120 μg/l (>0.99)	85.2–109.8 (<12)	0.18 to 0.62	0.60–2.08	[42]
20 mycotoxins	Grains	5 g sample, 25 ml ACN/H_2O (1% HOAc), 4 g $MgSO_4$, 1 g NaCl, 1 g of $Na_3Cit{\cdot}2H_2O$, and 0.5 g of $Na_2Cit{\cdot}1.5H_2O$	20 mg Fe_3O_4-MWCNTs, then filtered	UHPLC–MS/MS	1–500 (>0.99)	73.5–112.9 (1.3–12.7)	0.0006–1.6337	0.0021–5.4457	[43]
AF(B1, B2, G1, G2), OTA	Apple juice, raisin, wheat flour, peanut, spices	2–2.5 g sample, 10 ml ACN (1% HOAc), 7.5 ml of H_2O, 4 g $MgSO_4$, 1 g NaCl, 1 g of $Na_3Cit{\cdot}2H_2O$, and 0.5 g of $Na_2Cit{\cdot}1.5H_2O$	0.2 g PSA, 0.6 g $MgSO_4$.(low fat) 150 mg of C18, 900 mg $MgSO_4$ (high fat)	LC–MS/MS	1–30 (>0.996)	81.94–101.67 (0.12–10.28)	0.05–0.1	0.08–0.3	[44]
ZEA, T-2, AFB1, DON, OTA	Corn flour	5 g sample, 15 ml ACN/H_2O/HCOOH, 5 g $MgSO_4$, 1 g NaCl,	1 g $MgSO_4$ and 0.3 g PSA, dried +1 ml MeOH	LC–MS/MS	2–1800	92.9–103.8 (3.7–20)	2–75	0.6–25	[45]

Aflatoxins	Sample Matrix	QuEChERS procedure	Clean-Up method	Instrumental analysis	Linearity (μg/kg) (R^2)	Recovery (%) (RSD %)	LOD (μg/kg)	LOQ (μg/kg)	Reference
AF(B1, B2, G1, G2), T-2, HT-2	Cereal derived products	2 g sample, 10 ml H_2O (1% HOAC), 10 ml ACN, 4 g $MgSO_4$, 1 g NaCl,	2 ml extract evaporated +200 μl $MeOH/H_2O$, then filtered	LC–MS/MS	2–140 (>0.990)	83.8–102.9 (14.3–15.7)	0.5–100	1–200	[46]
ZEA, DON	Cereal	4 g sample, 16 ml ACN/H_2O, 6 g $MgSO_4$, 1.5 g NaCl, 1.5 g sodium citrate dehydrate, 1 g sodium citrate sesquihydrate	300 mg PSA, 100 mg $MgSO_4$, dried +1 ml of MeOH/PBS	ELISA	13.64–983.52 ng/ml ((n.r)		2.58–17.31 ng/ml	n.r	[47]
AF(B1, B2, G1, G2, M1, M2), OTA, OTB, ZEA	Egg	5 g sample, 5 ml Na_2EDTA, 20 ml of ACN (1% of HOAc), 4 g Na_2SO_4, 1 g NaCl	15 mg of Fe_3O_4-MWCNTs, separated by external magnetic field. 1 ml extract +1 ml $MeOH/H_2O$, filtered	UHPLC–MS/MS	1–100 (n.r)	71.8–100.0 (1.6–17.3)	n.r	0.2–11.8	[48]
26 mycotoxins	Sesame butter	2.5 g sample, 20 ml ACN/H_2O (0.1% HCOOH), 4 g $MgSO_4$, 1 g NaCl, 1 g sodium citrate, 0.5 g sodium hydrogen citrate sesquihydrate	150 mg C18, 900 mg $MgSO_4$,	UHPLC–MS/MS	0.5–500 ng/ml (>0.994)	48.70–111.70	0.05–7.25	0.11–21.74	[49]
AF(B1, B2, G1, G2), F (B1, B2, B3), ZEA, DON	Corn	2 g sample, 20 ml ACN/H_2O, 2 g $MgSO_4$, 0.5 g NaCl	30 mg C18	UPLC-Q-TOFMS	2.5–2000 (>0.991)	68.0–120.0 (0.18–6.29)	0.05–50	0.1–200	[50]

Aflatoxins	Sample Matrix	QuEChERS procedure	Clean-Up method	Instrumental analysis	Linearity (μg/kg) (R^2)	Recovery (%) (RSD %)	LOD (μg/kg)	LOQ (μg/kg)	Reference
14 mycotoxins	Rice	10 g sample, 4 g $MgSO_4$, 1 g NaCl 4 g, 1 g sodium citrate tribasic dihydrate and 0.5 g sodium citrate dibasic sesquihydrate	1.2 g $MgSO_4$, 0.25 g C18, 0.25 g Al-N	UHPLC–MS/MS	10–2500 (>0.99)	70–98.5 (<7.0)	0.5–15	1.7–50	[52]

Key: *RSD, relative standard deviation;* R^2*, correlation coefficient; n.r, not reported; LOQ, limit of quantitation; LOD, limit of detection; AF, aflatoxin, DON, deoxynivalenol; F, Fumonisin; OTA. Ochratoxin A, OTB, ochratoxin; ZEA, zearalenone; T-2, T-2 toxin; HT-2, HT-2 toxin; MeOH, methanol; ACN, acetonitrile, HCOOH, formic acid; HOAc, acetic acid; HPLC, high performance liquid chromatography; UHPLC, ultra-high performance liquid chromatography; MS, mass spectrometry; FLD, fluorescence detector; UV, ultraviolet; DAD, diode array detector; Q-TOF, quadruple time-of-flight; PSA, primary secondary amine; Al-N, aluminum nitride.*

Table 1.
Applications of QuEChERS techniques for the analysis of aflatoxins in food samples.

range of 2.4–4.6 and 6.9–20.1 μg/kg, respectively. Other mycotoxins were not detectable in peanut butter [49].

A fast analytical method for the simultaneous determination of 9 mycotoxins in corn using dSPE and ultra-performance liquid chromatography coupled to tandem quadruple time-of-flight mass spectrometry (UPLC-Q-TOFMS) was developed and validated by Wang et al. (2016). The corn samples (2.00 g ± 0.01 g) were accurately weighed in a 50-ml polypropylene tube. The samples were extracted with 20 ml of acetonitrile-water (84:16, v:v) containing 1% acetic acid, in an ultrasonic water bath for 20 min at room temperature. $MgSO_4$ (2 g) and NaCl (0.5 g) were added, and the tube was shaken vigorously for 1 min and then centrifuged 5000 rpm for 5 min. The supernatant was transferred to a separate centrifuge tube each containing C18 powder, PSA and GCB, (with 30 mg of C18 giving highest recovery) and shaken for 1 min and then centrifuged for 5 min at 5000 rpm. The supernatant was collected and then the tube was blown to near dryness under nitrogen. The pellet was redissolved with methanol–water and the solution was filtered through a 0.22 μm PTFE syringe filter and the filtrate was subjected to instrumental analysis. The mean recoveries were ranged from 68.0 to 120.0%, and the relative standard deviation (RSD) ranged from 0.18 to 6.29%. The linearity ranged from 2.5 to 2000 μg/kg with correlation coefficient greater than 0.99, while limits of detections ranged from 0.05 to 50 μg/kg, and limits of quantification ranged from 0.1 to 200 μg/kg, which were below the legal limits set by the European Union for the legislated mycotoxins. The developed method was applied to 130 corn samples. Among the mycotoxins studied, aflatoxins B1 and fumonisins B1, B2 and B3 were the most predominant mycotoxins, and their concentrations were 0–593.12, 0–2.01 × 104, 0–6.94 × 103 and 0–3.05 × 103 μg/kg, respectively [50].

A sample preparation based on QuEChERS was developed of the analysis of 14 mycotoxins in rice. The method involved mixing 10 g of rice sample with 10 ml of water and 10 ml of acetonitrile containing 10% formic acid. The mixture was then shake with automatic shaker followed by addition of 4 g $MgSO_4$, 1 g sodium citrate tribasic dihydrate and 0.5 g sodium citrate dibasic sesquihydrate and the tube was shaken vigorously with hand for 1 min, and then centrifuged for 5 min at 3400 rpm. The supernatant was transferred to dSPE tube containing 1.2 g of $MgSO_4$, 0.25 g of C18, 0.25 g of aluminum nitride and 0.4 g PSA and the tube was centrifuged at 3400 rpm for 5 min. The supernatant was evaporated to dryness under stream of nitrogen and was reconstituted with 1 ml of mixture of methanol/acetonitrile (1:1 v/v %), vortexed for 1 min and filtered through 0.2 um nylon syringe filter, and the filtrate was analyzed using ultra performance liquid chromatography triple quadruple mass spectrometer (UHPLC–MS/MS). The method validation gave linearity ranging from 10 to 2500 μg/kg with correlation coefficient greater than 0.99. The average recoveries ranged from 70 to 98.5% and RSD less than 7%. The LOQ and LOD were 1.7–50 μg/kg and 0.5–15 μg/kg, respectively. The developed method was validated according to the European Communities 2002/657/EC and SANCO/12495/2011 [51] guidelines and met acceptability criteria in all cases. The performance of the QuEChERS method was compared with the performance of commercial immuneaffinity column (IACs) and the IAC gave comparable performance, but with higher LODs compared to the developed QuEChERS method, but suffered from some limitations, such as lack of sensitivity for some mycotoxins, does not allow multi-analysis and possible cross-reactivity (**Table 1**) [52].

5. Conclusion

Mycotoxins are secondary fungi metabolites present in foods which can cause adverse effects on humans and animals. Therefore, it is essential to develop a simple, effective, sensitive and validated analytical method to monitor mycotoxins. Sample preparation is an important step in the analysis of mycotoxins and other contaminants from complex food matrices. And due to the growing demand for high-throughput multiresidue methods (MRM), researchers have developed several easy to perform sample treatment methods, which are rapid and of low cost, require a minimum volume of solvents, provide a high selectivity without complicated clean-up solutions, and allow analysis of broad range of analytes. QuEChERS is fast and simple analytical method which has been developed and optimized for the analysis of a fast and simple analytical method, although several researchers have over the years modified the original QuEChERS technique, which allow multiresidue analysis.

Most of the QuEChERS methods described in this review were couple to liquid chromatography analysis. This is partly due to the great increases in its sensitivity and selectivity, which has led to a significant contribution in qualitative and quantitative determination of mycotoxins in cereals and related foodstuffs. Also, the increasing use of hybrid mass spectrometers, incorporating mass analyzers that are capable of high mass resolution and accurate mass measurements, mitigates some of the problems associated with selectivity and identification. The improvement and upgrading of the available techniques will determine the effectiveness and efficiency of mycotoxins analysis in food matrices.

Author details

Lukman Bola Abdulra'uf[1*], Kikelomo Elizabeth Ayeni[1,2], Abdulrahman Ibraheem[1], Aisha Ishaq[1], Abibat Monisola Junaid[1,3], Mutiat Aliu[1], Abubakar Lawal[4] and Guan Huat Tan[5]

1 Faculty of Pure and Applied Science, Department of Chemistry and Industrial Chemistry, Kwara State University, Ilorin, Kwara State, Nigeria

2 Department of Science Laboratory Technology, Federal Polytechnic, Offa, Kwara State, Nigeria

3 Department of Chemistry, College of Sciences, Kwara State College of Education, Ilorin, Kwara State, Nigeria

4 Faculty of Natural and Applied Sciences, Department of Pure and Industrial Chemistry, Umaru Musa Yar'adua University, Kastina, Nigeria

5 Faculty of Science, Department of Chemistry, University of Malaya, Kuala Lumpur, Malaysia

*Address all correspondence to: abdulrauf.bola@kwasu.edu.ng

References

[1] Saleem F, Sadia B, Awan FS. Control of aflatoxin production using herbal plant extract. In: Abdulra'uf LB, editor. Aflatoxin-Control, Analysis, Detection and Health Risks. Rijeka: InTech; 2017. pp. 1-12

[2] Sirhan AY et al. QuEChERS-HPLC method for aflatoxin detection of domestic and imported food in JORDAN. Journal of Liquid Chromatography & Related Technologies. 2014;**37**(3):321-342

[3] Wacoo AP et al. Methods for detection of aflatoxins in agricultural food crops. Journal of Applied Chemistry. 2014;**2014**:706291

[4] FAO. In: Food and Agricultural Organization of the United Nations (FAO), editor. International Code of Conduct on Pesticide Management: Guideline on Pesticide Legislation. Rome: FAO; 2015

[5] Nikolas P et al. Occurence of mycotoxins and mycotoxicosis in poultry. Concept of Diary & Veterinary Sciences. 2018;**2**(1):165-167

[6] CAC. In: Codex Alimentarius Food Standard, editor. General Standard for Contaminants and Toxins in Food and Feed. Rome, Italy: FAO/WHO; 2017

[7] Zhang K, Banerjee K. A review: Sample preparation and chromatographic technologies for detection of aflatoxins in foods. Toxins. 2020;**12**(9):539

[8] Spanjer MC, Rensen PM, Scholten JM. LC-MS/MS multi-method for mycotoxins after single extraction, with validation data for peanut, pistachio, wheat, maize, cornflakes, raisins and figs. Food Additives & Contaminants. Part A, Chemistry, Analysis, Control, Exposure & Risk Assessment. 2008; **25**(4):472-489

[9] Turner C. Overview of modern extraction techniques for food and agricultural samples. In: Turner C, editor. Modern Extraction Techniques. Washington DC, USA: ACS; 2006. pp. 3-19

[10] Chavez RA, Cheng X, Stasiewicz MJ. A review of the methodology of Analyzing aflatoxin and fumonisin in single corn kernels and the potential impacts of these methods on food security. Food. 2020;**9**(3):297

[11] Abdulra'uf LB, Tan GH. Multivariate study of parameters in the determination of pesticide residues in apple by headspace solid phase microextraction coupled to gas chromatography–mass spectrometry using experimental factorial design. Food Chemistry. 2013; **141**(4):4344-4348

[12] Falaki F. In: Kusch P, editor. Sample preparation techniques for gas chromatography, Gas Chromatography Derivatization, Sample Preparation, Application. Rijeka: Intech Open; 2019

[13] Sharifi V, Abbasi A, Nosrati A. Application of hollow fiber liquid phase microextraction and dispersive liquid–liquid microextraction techniques in analytical toxicology. Journal of Food and Drug Analysis. 2016;**24**(2):264-276

[14] Abdulra'uf LB et al. Review of ionic liquids in microextraction analysis of pesticide residues in fruit and vegetable samples. Chromatographia. 2020;**83**: 11-33

[15] Anastassiades M et al. Fast and easy multiresidue method employing acetonitrile extraction/partitioning and

"dispersive solid-phase extraction" for the determination of pesticide residues in produce. Journal of Association of Official Analytical Chemists International. 2003;**86**(2):412-431

[16] Casado N, Morante-Zarcero S, Sierra I. Application of the QuEChERS strategy as a useful sample preparation tool for the multiresidue determination of pyrrolizidine alkaloids in food and feed samples: A critical overview. Applied Sciences. 2022;**12**(9):4325

[17] Lehotay SJ et al. Comparison of QuEChERS sample preparation methods for the analysis of pesticide residues in fruits and vegetables. Journal of Chromatography. A. 2010;**1217**: 2548-2560

[18] Musarurwa H, Chimuka L, Tavengwa NT. Green pre-concentration techniques during pesticide analysis in food samples. Journal of Environmental Science and Health. Part. B. 2019;**54**(9): 770-780

[19] Anastassiades M et al. In: Ohkawa H, Miyagawa H, Lee PW, editors. Recent developments in QuEChERS methodology for pesticide multiresidue analysis, Pesticide Chemistry: Crop Protection. Public Health, Environmental Safety. Japan: WILEY-ICH; 2007:439-458

[20] Rodríguez-Carrasco Y et al. Simultaneous determination of AFB1 and AFM1 in milk samples by ultra high performance liquid chromatography coupled to quadrupole orbitrap mass spectrometry. Beverages. 2018; **4**(2):43

[21] Gotah A, Whang K, Garcia CV. Determination of aflatoxins in rice using QuEChERS and fluorescence HPLC. Scientific Study and Research. 2018; **19**(2):133-141

[22] Gong X et al. Determination of 15 mycotoxins in foods and feeds using high performance liquid chromatography-tandem mass spectrometry with gel permeation chromatography combined QuEChERS purification. Journal of Chromatography & Separation Techniques. 2012;**3**:1-7

[23] Miró-Abella E et al. Determination of mycotoxins in plant-based beverages using QuEChERS and liquid chromatography-tandem mass spectrometry. Food Chemistry. 2017; **229**:366-372

[24] Azaiez I et al. Multi-mycotoxins analysis in dried fruit by LC/MS/MS and a modified QuEChERS procedure. Food Analytical Methods. 2014;**7**(4): 935-945

[25] Cunha SC, Sá SVM, Fernandes JO. Multiple mycotoxin analysis in nut products: Occurrence and risk characterization. Food and Chemical Toxicology. 2018;**114**:260-269

[26] Eissa AA, Hassan ASM, El-Rahman TMA. Determination of total aflatoxins and carbamate pesticide residues in some bee honey samples using QuEChERS method and high performance liquid chromatography. Food and Public Health. 2014;**4**:209-213

[27] Bursic VP et al. Analysis of aflatoxins B1 and G1 in maize by QUEChERS. Matica Srpska Journal for Natural Sciences. 2013;**124**:51-57

[28] Sartori A et al. Determination of aflatoxins M1, M2, B1, B2, G1, and G2 and ochratoxin a in UHT and powdered Milk by modified QuEChERS method and ultra-high-performance liquid chromatography tandem mass spectrometry. Food Analytical Methods. 2015;**8**:2321-2330

[29] Jettanajit A, Nhujak T. Determination of mycotoxins in brown rice using QuEChERS sample preparation and UHPLC-MS-MS. Journal of Chromatographic Science. 2016;**54**(5): 720-729

[30] IAL. Métodos fisicoquímicos para análise de alimentos: micotoxinas. Sao Paulo: Instituto Adolfo Lutz; 2008

[31] Sirhan AY, Tan GH, Wong RCS. Method validation in the determination of aflatoxins in noodle samples using the QuEChERS method (quick, easy, cheap, effective, rugged and safe) and high performance liquid chromatography coupled to a fluorescence detector (HPLC-FLD). Food Control. 2011;**22**:1807-1813

[32] EU. Commission regulation EC n. 401/2006 of 23 February 2006. Laying down the methods of sampling and analysis for the official control of the levels of mycotoxins in foodstuffs. Official Journal of the European Union. 2006;**70**:12-34

[33] Trombete F et al. In-house validation of a method for determining aflatoxins B1, B2, G1 and G2 in wheat and wheat by-products. Pesquisa Agropecuária Tropical. 2014;**44**:255-262

[34] Pantano L et al. QuEChERS LC–MS/MS screening method for mycotoxin detection in cereal products and spices. International Journal of Environmental Research and Public Health. 2021;**18**:3774

[35] Choochuay S et al. Determination of aflatoxin B 1 in feedstuffs without clean-up step by high-performance liquid chromatography. International Journal of Analytical Chemistry. 2018;**2018**:1-8

[36] Karaseva N, Amelin V, Tretyakov AV. QuEChERS coupled to dispersive liquid–liquid microextraction for the determination of aflatoxins B1 and M1 in dairy foods by HPLC. Journal of Analytical Chemistry. 2014;**69**(5):510-515

[37] Sartori A et al. Determination of aflatoxins M1, M2, B1, B2, G1 and G2 in peanut by modified QuEChERS method and ultra-high performance liquid chromatography-tandem mass spectrometry. Vigilância Sanitária em Debate. 2014;**3**:115-121

[38] Desmarchelier A et al. Development and comparison of two multiresidue methods for the analysis of 17 mycotoxins in cereals by liquid chromatography electrospray ionization tandem mass spectrometry. Journal of Agricultural and Food Chemistry. 2010; **58**(13):7510-7519

[39] Dos Anjos MR et al. Multiresidue method for simultaneous analysis of aflatoxin M1, avermectins, organophosphate pesticides and milbemycin in milk by ultra-performance liquid chromatography coupled to tandem mass spectrometry. Food Additives & Contaminants. Part A, Chemistry, Analysis, Control, Exposure & Risk Assessment. 2016;**33**(6):995-1002

[40] Jo H-W et al. Simultaneous determination of 13 mycotoxins in feedstuffs using QuEChERS extraction. Applied Biological Chemistry. 2021; **64**(1):34

[41] Zhao H et al. Determination of 16 mycotoxins in vegetable oils using a QuEChERS method combined with high-performance liquid chromatography-tandem mass spectrometry. Food Additives & Contaminants. Part A, Chemistry, Analysis, Control, Exposure & Risk Assessment. 2017;**34**(2):255-264

[42] Sirhan AY, Tan GH, Wong RCS. QuEChERS extraction and HPLC-FLD determination of ochratoxin a in cereals

and cereal products. Asian Journal of Chemistry. 2012;**22**:4551-4554

[43] Ma S et al. Using magnetic multiwalled carbon nanotubes as modified QuEChERS adsorbent for simultaneous determination of multiple mycotoxins in grains by UPLC-MS/MS. Journal of Agricultural and Food Chemistry. 2019;**67**(28):8035-8044

[44] Alsharif AMA, Choo Y-M, Tan G-H. Detection of five mycotoxins in different food matrices in the Malaysian market by using validated liquid chromatography electrospray ionization triple quadrupole mass spectrometry. Toxins. 2019;**11**(4):196

[45] Amirahmadi M et al. Simultaneous analysis of mycotoxins in corn flour using LC/MS-MS combined with a modified QuEChERS procedure. Toxin Reviews. 2018;**37**(3):187-195

[46] Annunziata L et al. Simultaneous determination of aflatoxins, T-2 and HT-2 toxins, and fumonisins in cereal-derived products by QuEChERS extraction coupled with LC-MS/MS. Analytical and Bioanalytical Chemistry. 2017;**409**(21):5143-5155

[47] He Q et al. QuEChERS extraction followed by enzyme-linked immunosorbent assay for determination of deoxynivalenol and zearalenone in cereals. Food and Agricultural Immunology. 2017;**28**(6):1477-1495

[48] Xu X et al. Development of a modified QuEChERS method based on magnetic multiwalled carbon nanotubes for the simultaneous determination of veterinary drugs, pesticides and mycotoxins in eggs by UPLC-MS/MS. Food Chemistry. 2019;**276**:419-426

[49] Liu Y et al. Modified QuEChERS method combined with ultra-high performance liquid chromatography tandem mass spectrometry for the simultaneous determination of 26 mycotoxins in sesame butter. Journal of Chromatography. B, Analytical Technologies in the Biomedical and Life Sciences. 2014;**970**:68-76

[50] Wang Y et al. Fast determination of multi-mycotoxins in corn by dispersive solid-phase extraction coupled with ultra-performance liquid chromatography with tandem quadrupole time-of-flight mass spectrometry. Journal of Integrative Agriculture. 2016;**15**(7):1656-1666

[51] SANCO. In: European Union, editor. Method Validation and Quality Control Procedures for Pesticide Residues Analysis in Food and Feed; Brussel: SANCO/12495/2011; 2011

[52] Koesukwiwat U, Sanguankaew K, Leepipatpiboon N. Evaluation of a modified QuEChERS method for analysis of mycotoxins in rice. Food Chemistry. 2014;**153**:44-51

Chapter 7

Aflatoxin B_1: An Immunomodulator and Cancer Agent

Mohamed Mutocheluh and Patrick Williams Narkwa

Abstract

The type I interferon signaling pathway of the innate immune system plays a key role in the first line of defense in eliminating pathogens and other chemical agents that are introduced into the body and is also known to exhibit the anticancer properties. Therefore, any agent being chemical or components of microorganisms that tend to inhibit or suppress the type I interferon response pathway will weaken the innate immune system and predispose individuals to infectious agents and cancers. Aflatoxin B_1 has been reported to modulate the immune system by suppressing inflammatory cytokines, monocytes, lymphocytes and the type I interferon signaling response pathway. Aflatoxin B_1 contamination of food is very high in most sub-Saharan African countries. Aflatoxin B_1 contamination of diet coupled with subsequent prolonged heavy exposure is one of the major risk factors for the development of hepatocellular carcinoma. Aflatoxin B_1 is known to cause hepatocellular carcinoma by inducing mutation in the tumor suppressor gene TP53. We present in this review the mechanism by which aflatoxin B_1 inhibits the type I interferon signaling pathway thus pre-disposing exposed individuals to cancers and other infections.

Keywords: aflatoxin B_1, hepatocellular carcinoma, cancer, immunosuppression, type I interferon, hepatocarcinogen

1. Introduction

Aflatoxins (AFBs) are mycotoxins that were discovered in the 1960s when 120,000 turkeys and poultry birds fed with poultry feed imported from South America died of Turkey X disease in England [1]. *Aspergillus parasiticus* and *Aspergillus flavus* are the two most common species of the genus *Aspergillus* that are known to biosynthesize aflatoxins. Chemically, aflatoxins are secondary metabolites that is they are substances that are made by living agents which do not need them for their survival. In relation to their chemical structure, AFBs consist of bifuran ring that is fused to a coumarins ring. Twenty (20) different metabolites of AFBs have been currently discovered. The most important AFBs out of the 20 currently discovered ones are aflatoxin B_1 (AFB_1), aflatoxin B_2 (AFB_2), aflatoxin G_1 (AFG_1) and aflatoxin G_2 (AFG_2).

Out of the different varieties of AFBs discovered, AFB_1 is reported to be the commonest contaminant of food stuffs such as groundnut and maize that are heavily consumed by many Africans and is considered the most lethal carcinogen in humans [2, 3]. The International Agency for Research on Cancer (IARC) has classified AFB_1

IntechOpen

as group 1 human carcinogen [4]. It is estimated that about 4.5 billion people worldwide are persistently exposed to food stuffs contaminated with aflatoxins. In many developing countries including Ghana, most people rely heavily on maize, groundnut and other types of cereals as their staple food which are invariably contaminated with AFB_1. In countries like Ghana, Benin and Togo which are located in West Africa, it has been reported that some food stuffs meant for human consumption contain high levels of AFBs [5–7]. The reasons for the high level of AFB_1 in these foods are due to poor storage conditions, high humidity in the West African sub region as well as suboptimal farming practices. Weanimix, a local food made from maize and groundnut in Ghana has been reported to contain high level of AFBs above the national acceptable level of 15ppb [8]. Prolonged heavy consumption of diet contaminated with AFB_1 is a significant risk factor that can cause hepatocellular carcinoma (HCC) [9, 10]. In addition to prolonged AFB_1 exposure, chronic infections with hepatitis B and C viruses (HBV; HCV), iron overload and excessive alcohol consumption have been identified as other factors of the environment that can cause HCC [11]. It has been reported that every year approximately 550,000 to 600,000 new HCC cases are recorded globally and that 25,200 to 155,000 are induced by AFBs exposure with majority of AFBs induced HCC cases occurring China, Southeastern part of Asia and West Africa [12].

Even though AFB_1 has serious negative effects in the human system, the type I interferon signaling response pathway of the innate immune system continually work in protecting individuals against disease causing agents and the harmful effects of AFBs. The type I interferon signaling response pathway plays a key role in eliminating disease causing microorganisms such as viruses as well as cancer cells. A study conducted to determine the capability of interferon to change back the phenotypic characteristics of tumor cells to normal phenotype reported that interferon was able to partially reverse phenotype of the tumorigenic cells in human osteosarcoma cells [13].

In 1986, Food and Drug Administration (FDA) of United States of America (USA) sanctioned the use of interferon-alpha 2a and 2b to treat Kaposi sarcoma in AIDS patients, cancer of the bone marrow (hairy cell leukemia) and other cancers [14]. Interferon treatment has been reported to activate p53, an anti-oncogene that plays a significant role in programmed cancer cell death [14]. Additionally, interferon-alpha has been reported to exhibit a significant protective effect against hepatic carcinogenesis as well as fibrogenesis [15]. Aziz et al. [15] treated liver cells of rat with carcinogenic compounds carbon tetrachloride and AFB_1 and revealed that cirrhotic and fibrotic processes in cells that were able to express ectopic IFN-α were minimized. Even though the experiment conducted by Aziz et al. [15] has not been replicated in the liver cells of human to evaluate the ability of viruses to induce the production of IFN in cases where individuals have been exposed to AFB_1, it demonstrated that interferon-alpha is a major protective agent against liver cancer. In this review, we present the mechanisms by which AFB_1 suppresses the type I interferon signaling response pathway thus predisposing individuals exposed to AFB_1 to cancers and other infections.

2. Distribution of fungi that produce aflatoxins

Aflatoxins are synthesized in food crops by two main fungal agents namely *Aspergillus parasiticus* and *Aspergillus flavus*. Even though the geographical locations of both *Aspergillus parasiticus* and *Aspergillus flavus* are similar, *Aspergillus parasiticus* is uncommon in Southeastern region of Asia. However, *Aspergillus flavus* is found everywhere predominantly in cereals that are grown in environment with low water condition and high temperature. *Aspergillus parasiticus* and *Aspergillus flavus* are mostly found in food crops like groundnuts, maize, peanuts, spices, oilseeds, walnuts, millet, almonds, corn, cottonseed, corn, and others. *Aspergillus flavus* and *Aspergillus parasiticus* predominantly produce AFB_1 and AFB_2 during growth periods, when crops are being harvested, threshed, dried, stored and transported [16]. *Aspergillus parasiticus* predominantly produce AFG_1 and AFG_2 [16]. *Aspergillus nomius, Aspergillus australis, Aspergillus fumigatus* and *Aspergillus niger* are other species of *Aspergillus* which produce AFBs. *Aspergillus* species mainly colonize the soil, decaying organic matter, grains and hay that are deteriorating microbiologically. *Aspergillus species* grow and produce AFBs in an environment that is moist and hot [17].

3. Types of aflatoxins, structure and properties of AFB_1

To date twenty (20) different types of AFBs have been discovered. Of these 20 currently known AFBs, the major ones include AFB_1, AFB_2, AFG_1, AFG_2, aflatoxin M_1 (AFM_1) and aflatoxin M_2 (AFM_2). The AFB_1, AFB_2, AFG_1 and AFG_2 are made by fungi while AFM_1 and AFM_2 are made as intermediate products when AFB_1 and AFB_2 respectively are metabolized. The B and G descriptions of AFBs refer to the type of color generated when AFBs are placed under short-wave UV (ultraviolet) illumination during thin layer chromatography. The B description of AFB_1 and AFB_2 refers to the blue light generated under UV illumination while the G description refers to the green light generated under UV illumination on thin layer chromatographic plates. The AFM_1 and AFM_2 were initially detected in raw milk of livestock that had ingested feed contaminated with AFBs thus the description M. The subscript numbers 1 and 2 indicate the major and minor compounds respectively [18–20].

Structurally, AFB_1 like all other AFBs consist of bifuran ring that is fused to a coumarins ring. AFB molecules differ from AFG molecules in that AFB molecules have cyclopentenone ring while the AFG molecules have lactone ring. There are double bonds at loci 8 and 9 on the terminal furan ring of the AFB_1 structure and these double bonds confer the unique carcinogenic characteristics to AFB_1 (**Figure 1**) [21].

Generally, AFBs occur as crystals which appear as uncolored or lemon-yellow at 25 to 28°C [22]. AFBs are partially soluble in water and hydrocarbons but cannot be dissolved in hydrophobic solvents. AFBs are completely dissolvable in polar solvent like alcohol (e.g. methanol), acetone and chloroform. To degrade AFBs, they can be placed in light and air. AFBs can also be degraded by exposing them to UV light,

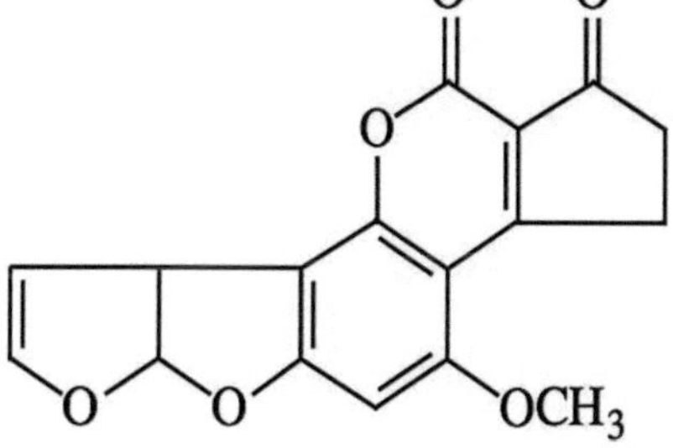

Figure 1.
Chemical structure of AFB_1.

strong acid solution, strong basic solution and oxidizing agents. AFBs can be broken down by exposing them to very high temperature conditions ranging between 237 to 299°C. Complete destruction of AFBs can be achieved when they are autoclaved with ammonia or when they are treated with bleach containing sodium hypochlorite. Normal cooking temperatures cannot degrade AFBs.

4. Biotransformation of aflatoxins

Metabolism of AFB_1 largely occurs in the liver by a group of enzymes called cytochrome P450 (CYP 450). When AFB_1 is ingested, it is transported to the liver where the CYP 450 enzymes convert AFB_1into different compounds which include AFM_1, aflatoxicol, aflatoxin P_1 (AFP_1) and aflatoxin Q_1 (AFQ_1). Additionally, the CYP450 enzymes especially CYP1A2 and CYP3A4 convert AFB_1 into reactive oxygen species (ROS) AB_1–8, 9-epoxide which exists in two (2) forms; endo-AFB_1–8, 9-epoxide and exo-AB_1–8, 9-epoxide. Whereas the CYP3A4 produces exo-AB_1–8, 9-epoxide and a small quantity of AFQ_1, the CYP1A2 produces both endo and exo-AFB_1–8, 9-epoxides as well as AFM_1 [23]. Of the two epoxide species, exo-AFB_1–8, 9-epoxide is considered to be the toxic species that confers genotoxic characteristics on AFB_1 [2, 3, 24]. The AFB_1–8, 9 epoxide metabolites formed can form conjugates with glutathione leading to the formation of a stable, harmless, soluble product which is excreted in the bile. The conjugation process is catalyzed by the enzyme glutathione-S-transferase (GST). The conjugation and the subsequent excretion of the soluble product formed is the mechanism by which AFB_1 is detoxified as a hepatocarcinogen. The AFB_1–8, 9 epoxide-glutathione complex formed is also broken down in the liver and kidney is excreted in the urine as mercapturic acid [25]. On the other hand, when individuals are exposed to high levels of AFB_1 beyond the capability of GST enzymes to break down the epoxides into harmless forms, or when the activity of GST enzymes is reduced through

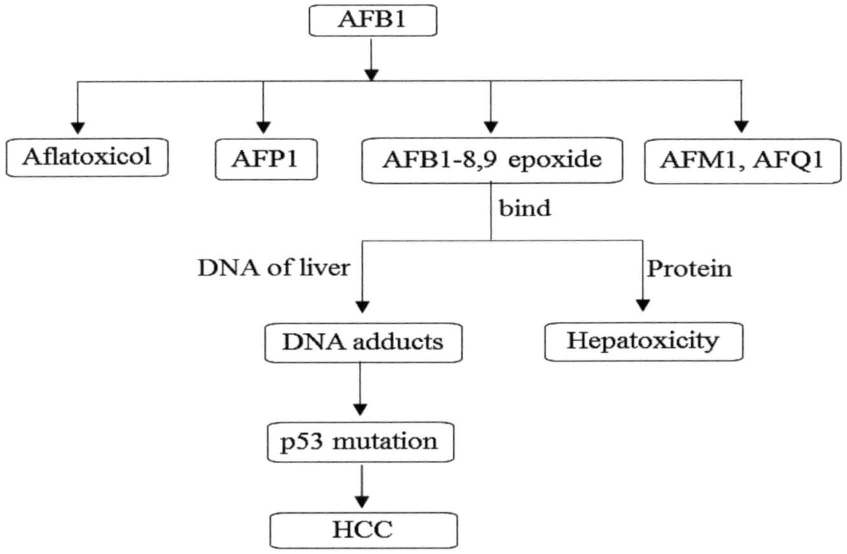

Figure 2.
Schematic flow chart on metabolism of AFB_1.

mutations of the GST gene, the AFB_1–8, 9 epoxides can bind to liver proteins and cause their failure which can result in acute hepatotoxicity or aflatoxicosis.

Conversely, the 8, 9 epoxides can cause mutations of DNA in the liver cells and as a results pro-mutagenic lesions may be formed. When the pro-mutagenic lesions are formed, proto-oncogenes are activated and this may cause the tumor suppressor genes to become inactivated. The AFB_1–8, 9 epoxide has affinity for the N^7 atom of guanine and so bind with it which leads to the production of a pro-mutagenic DNA adduct (AFB_1-N^7-Gua adduct). The AFB_1-N^7-Gua adduct is not stable and so goes through depurination process which results in the adduct being excreted in the urine. Animals such as mice that are more immune to the carcinogenic effects of AFB_1 have much greater GST action compared to animals such as rats which more susceptible to the carcinogenic effects of AFB_1. In humans, the action of GST enzymes is much lower when compared with rats and mice. This suggests that the ability of humans to detoxify AFB_1–8, 9 epoxides is lower [26] and therefore humans stand a greater chance of suffering from the carcinogenic effects of AFB_1 when compared with rats and mice. **Figure 2** below shows the schematic flow chart on how metabolism of AFB_1 occurs in the liver.

5. Effects of aflatoxins on human health

AFBs are very genotoxic agents that can still cause ailment in human beings when individuals are exposed to small quantities [27]. Even though AFBs can cause disease in many parts of the human system, they are largely known to cause acute and or chronic disease in the liver as well as liver cancer. There are so many ways by which AFBs manifest their toxic side effects when ingested into the body. AFBs can modify the integrity of the intestines [28] and regulate the expression of cytokines. These negative effects of AFBs can lead to impaired growth and weakening of the immune system in children [29]. The quantity or amount of AFBs consumed or ingested coupled with how long the individual has been exposed largely determine the negative impact of AFBs in humans and other animals. Acute exposure of humans to AFBs occur when large amount of AFBs are consumed within shortest possible time. Chronic exposure occurs when humans consume minute quantities of AFBs over a prolonged period of time.

When humans are exposed to large quantities of AFBs over a relatively short time period, it can results in vomiting, stomach aches, mental retardation, improper digestion of food, liver disease, coma and hepatotoxicity or aflatoxicosis. About 25% of individuals who experience acute AFBs exposure die from AFBs-related diseases [30]. There are environmental factors which predispose humans to acute aflatoxicosis. These factors are scarcity of food, high temperatures and humid environment which promotes the growth of the fungi that produce AFBs and inadequate systems to regulate and monitor food stuffs for the presence AFBs. Globally acute aflatoxicosis has become a recurrent public health problem [31, 32].

Research indicates that prolong exposure of individuals to small quantities of AFBs can cause impairment of the immune system, reduction in absorption of nutrients from the small intestines which may ultimately result in stunted growth especially in children and young infants [33, 34]. Reports from research conducted within Togo as well as Benin, countries located in the West African sub-region indicate that there is a correlation between levels of AFB-protein (albumin) adduct and growth impairment [35, 36]. In 2005 Jiang et al. [37] undertook a study in Ghana and reported that individuals who had higher levels of AFB_1-albumin adducts had reduced levels of certain leukocytes types. Similarly, Turner et al. [38] undertook a study in Gambia and reported that infants who had high levels of aflatoxin-albumin adducts had lower quantities of IgA antibodies in their saliva.

6. Immunomodulatory effects of AFB_1 in humans

Data or information on how AFBs and the related compounds regulate the immune system is scanty. Reports indicate that AFBs and other mycotoxins can suppress the immune system through the inhibition of DNA replication, transcription and translation of genes that are required to switch on the innate and acquired immune system response by using myriad of mechanisms [39]. Studies have indicated that the AFB_1–8, 9-exo-epoxide that is formed when AFB_1 is metabolized reacts with DNA found in the mitochondria rather than with DNA found in the nucleus of the cell and this hinders the synthesis of ATP [40, 41]. The binding of the AFB_1–8, 9-exo-epoxide to DNA of the mitochondria results in the formation AFB_1-mitochondrial DNA adduct which leads to mutations in the membranes causing ballooning of the cell as well as disrupting the production of ATP [40, 42].

Studies have reported that AFB_1 and its intermediate products inhibit translation when they bind to important enzymes that are needed in the translation of mRNAs into proteins. AFB_1 and its intermediate products also suppress translation by blocking the activities of translocase in ribosomes and this suppress translation [43]. Additionally, it has been reported that aflatoxins negatively affect protein synthesis by interfering with substrates and enzymes that are needed for initiation, transcription and translation [44].

Furthermore, several research works have looked at how AFB_1 inhibit the immune system in humans. In 2015, Jiang et al. conducted a study to evaluate how the regulation of some pro-inflammatory cytokines such as IL-2, IL-4, IL-6, IL-10, IL-17, IFN-γ and TNF-α in the bowels of broiler birds could be affected by AFB_1. They reported that the transcript levels of the studied pro-inflammatory cytokines in broiler birds treated with AFB_1 were much lower than the levels in broiler birds that were not treated with AFB_1. Furthermore, Jiang et al. indicated that broiler birds that were treated with AFB_1 exhibited reduced amount of T-cells in the intestines in comparison with broiler birds that were not treated. Several studies have also reported the suppression or inhibition of transcription and translation of IL-4, IL-6 and IL-10 genes respectively by AFB_1in the peritoneal macrophages, splenic lymphocytes and macrophage cell lines [45–47].

On the contrarily, a study conducted by Li et al. [48] indicated that broiler birds that were fed with livestock feed containing 0.074 mg/kg showed an increase in the levels of IL-6, IFN-γ and TNF-α mRNA and protein expression in the spleen and serum. In 2014, Qian et al. [49] undertook a study to determine the impact of AFB_1 on the splenic lymphocyte phenotypes and the inflammatory cytokine production in male F344 rats. They indicated that rats that were exposed to AFB_1 showed a dose-dependent reduction in the level of IL-4 produced by $CD4^+$ T cells. Also Bruneau et al. [50] reported that AFB_1 induced the suppression or inhibition of IFN-γ and TNF-α expression by $CD4^+$T cells and $CD3^-$CD8a NK cells respectively. Bruneau et al. [45] in addition indicated that murine macrophages that were exposed to AFB_1 *in vitro* showed a reduction in the level of anti-inflammatory cytokine IL-10 but rather increased the level of pro-inflammatory cytokine IL-6. Taken together these studies suggest aflatoxins are immunosuppressive agents.

A study was conducted by Forouharmehr, Harkinezhad [50] to determine the impact of AFB_1 on how the expression of STAT5A can be affected by treating bovine mammary epithelial cells with AFB_1 and quantifying the mRNA levels of STAT5A using RT-qPCR. They indicated that cells that were treated with AFB_1 showed a great decline in the mRNA levels of STAT5A in a dose-dependent manner. They further reported that the suppression of the mRNA levels of STAT5A minimized the proliferation and differentiation of mammary epithelial cells, thus affecting the amount and the quality of milk protein that is produced.

In 1999, Rossano et al. [51] treated human monocytes that have been activated with lipopolysaccharide of bacteria with 0.01–1.0 pg/mL of AFB_1 in order to determine how AFB_1 could affect the expression and release of IL-1α, IL-6α, TNF-α. They reported that at 0.05 pg/mL of AFB_1, the levels of IL-1α, IL-6α, and TNF-α were greatly reduced and that AFB_1 totally shut off the transcription of their mRNAs. Rossano et al. further reported that transcript levels of β-actin remained unchanged by AFB_1. These findings made the researchers to make a conclusion that AFB_1 exerts it effects on the expression of cytokines likely by suppressing the transcription of certain mRNAs without affecting translation.

The type I interferon signaling response pathway of the innate immune system plays a significant part in eliminating disease causing microorganisms and cancer cells in the human system. The type I interferons exhibit antiviral as well as anti-cancer properties. The anti-cancer activities of type I interferon led to their use to treat cancers such as Kaposi sarcoma in AIDS patients, cancer of the bone marrow (hairy cell leukemia) and other forms of cancers [14]. In 1979, Hahon et al. [52] conducted a study to determine how AFB_1 could affect the induction of interferon production in monkey kidney cells (LLC-MK) that had been infected with influenza virus. They reported that AFB_1 inhibited influenza viral induction of interferon dose-dependently.

In other to understand the mechanism of AFB_1 inhibition of the interferon signaling response pathway, Narkwa et al., demonstrated in a study that AFB_1 suppressed IFN-α induced ISRE (interferon stimulated response element) signaling in a dose dependent manner using luciferase reporter gene assay (**Figure 3**), [53]. Further using RT-qPCR Narkwa et al. [53] showed that AFB_1 inhibits transcript expression levels of key signaling elements such as STAT1, JAK1 and OAS3 genes of the JAK–STAT-ISRE arm of the type 1 IFN response pathway. Some studies have reported that post-transcriptional processes may be involved in the translation of mRNA into protein [54]. This suggests that low mRNA expression may not directly results in lower expression of protein and oppositely. Consequently, after demonstrating that AFB_1 suppresses the transcript expression levels of STAT1, JAK1 and OAS3, Western blot assay was used to determine whether the suppression of transcript expression level of STAT1 by AFB_1 would ultimately affect its translation into protein. The authors observed that AFB_1 suppressed the translation of STAT1 mRNA into protein. The type I IFN signaling has been reported to exert its anti-cancer and antiviral response through the activation of the JAK–STAT-ISRE arm of the pathway (**Figure 4**) [53]. One component of the JAK–STAT-ISRE signaling pathway considered to have tumor suppressor function is STAT1 [55]. When activated, STAT1 suppresses tumor development by inducing programmed cell death [56] and also inhibit tumor maturation or growth [57]. Therefore the suppression/inhibition of STAT1 by AFB_1 as demonstrated by Narkwa et al., would definitely weaken the capacity of STAT1 to coordinate the expression of multitude of genes necessary to stimulate programmed cell death, prohibit multiplication and maturation of cells in response to AFB_1. Therefore, the above stated studies provide overwhelming evidence that aflatoxins in general and

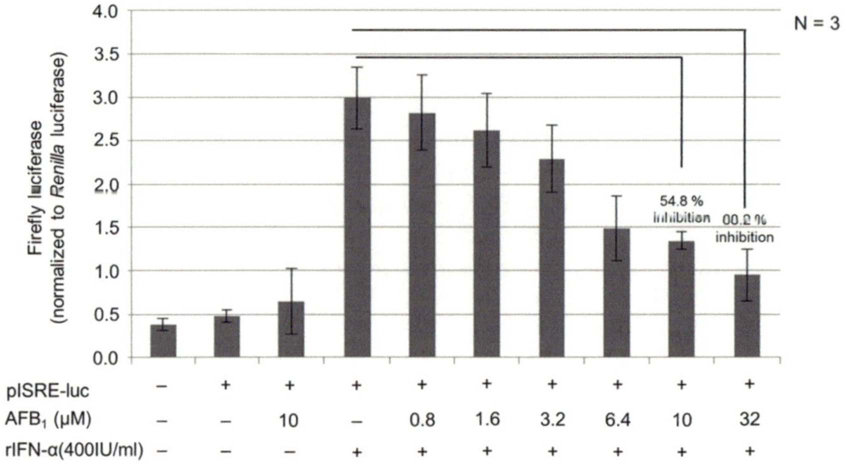

Figure 3.
AFB_1 suppresses the antiviral and anticancer type I interferon response signaling in a dose dependent manner. Source: [34].

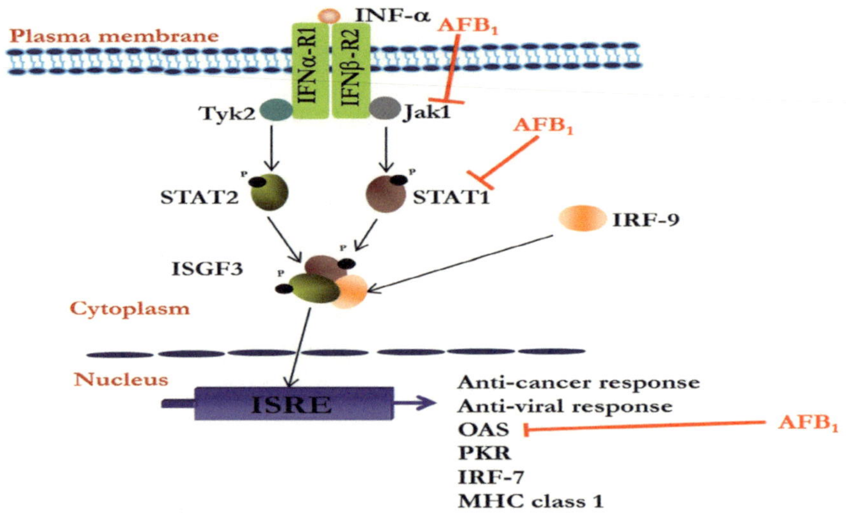

Figure 4.
Key antiviral and anticancer elements of the innate immune type I interferon signaling response pathway suppressed by AFB_1. Source: [34].

AFB_1 in particular suppress the immune system and predispose individuals to diseases including cancers.

7. AFB_1 as a cancer agent

As stated above, humans get exposed to AFB_1 when they consume food contaminated with aflatoxins or when they inhale dust particles containing aflatoxins and this could lead to acute or chronic aflatoxicosis. The signs and symptoms of aflatoxicosis include stomach ache, regurgitation, pulmonary congestion, multifocal hepatic necrosis and non-alcoholic fatty pancreatic disease. Again, AFB_1 is the major potent lethal human hepatocarcinogen and is classified as group 1 human carcinogen by the IARC [4] Data from Global Cancer Observatory Report (GLOBOCAN 2020) indicate that the global incidence of cancers in 2020 was roughly 19.3 million with 10 million cancer deaths. Cancer is reported as the leading cause of premature deaths globally [58]. The global rise of the cancers as leading cause of mortality resulted in the decline of both communicable and non-communicable diseases among humans.

HCC is the sixth commonest diagnosed cancer and the third leading cause of cancer mortality globally according to global cancer statistics 2020 report. HCC is more prevalent in resource limited countries. The most important factors that put individuals at risk of developing HCC comprise persistent HBV and HCV infections, AFB_1 exposure, excessive intake of alcohol and iron overload [11]. Aflatoxins particularly AFB_1 are established risk factors of HCC in humans and animals. In a case–control study to determine the association between aflatoxins and HCC, the authors reported that the average aflatoxin exposure per day in cases of HCC was 4.5 times higher than in the control groups [59]. A similar study in Mozambique directly correlated high dietary intake of aflatoxins to incidence of HCC [60]. Importantly, in the context of AFB_1 and HBV infection co-existing, the risk of developing HCC is increased by more than 30 times [61] compared to either HBV or aflatoxin exposure alone.

8. Mechanism of carcinogenesis of AFB_1

AFB_1 is a known genotoxic hepatocarcinogen that causes genetic damage such as formation of DNA adducts, albumin adduct, gene mutations, micronucleus formation, sister chromatid exchange and mitotic recombination which result in genetic changes in the target cells, which then cause DNA damage and ultimately cancer [26].

When AFB_1 is ingested by humans and other susceptible animals, it is transported to the liver where the CYP 450 enzymes convert AFB_1 into ROS endo-AFB_1–8, 9-epoxide and exo-AB_1–8, 9-epoxide the latter being more toxic than former, thus this confers genotoxic characteristics on AFB_1 [62]. The exo-AFB_1–8, 9 epoxide has affinity for the N^7 atom of guanine and so bind with it leading to the formation of primary DNA adduct (AFB_1-N^7-Gua adduct) [63]. The AFB_1-N^7-Gua adduct is transformed into two minor compounds namely an apurinic (AP) site and a stable ring-opened AFB_1-Formamidopyrimidine (AFB_1-FAPY) adduct the latter being more mutagenic than the former [21]. The AP and AFB_1-FAPY adduct are mended by nucleotide excision repair (NER) or base excision repair (BER) [64, 65].

Conversely, when the mending process is improperly done, it results in AGG to AGT transversion mutations with these mutations taking place at codon 249 in the tumor suppressor gene *TP53*. When these mutations occur, the amino acid arginine in the tumor suppressor protein p53 become replaced with serine (R249S) [66, 67]. When the mutated R249S p53 is expressed, apoptosis is inhibited, p53 mediated transcription is also inhibited and liver cells are stimulated to grow uncontrollably resulting in HCC [68]. Studies have reported that the R249S mutation is mostly found in more than 50% of HCC cases especially in China and Africa where the incidence of HCC is high [66, 69]. On the other hand, the R249S mutation is rare in the regions of the world where aflatoxins exist at extremely low levels in the diet and in cancers other than HCC [70]. The TP53 directs the synthesis of p53 protein. When the conditions within the cells are normal, the p53 is kept at low levels through it binding to ubiquitin-ligases such as Mdm2 (also referred to as Hdm2 in humans) and then degraded by proteasome enzymes [71]. On the other hand, in the presence of some stress factors, the p53 goes through certain processes such as phosphorylation on serine 15 (Pser15-p53) and become activated after it has been produced. The activated p53 binds specific DNA response elements resulting in trans-activation of genes that play key roles in programmed cell death, the arrest of cell cycle, repair of DNA repair or aging [72]. These responses lead to repair of damage that have been caused to DNA which help to maintain the genetic integrity of the cells. The response may also stimulate apoptosis of damaged cells resulting in their elimination from the system.

Some studies reported that AFB_1 impair miRNA biogenesis; the authors also reported that AFB_1 suppress Wnt/β-catenin signaling pathway by inducing over-expression of miR-34a and thus causing liver cancer [73]. Other studies showed that AFB_1 promote HCC cell multiplication through an IGF-2-dependent signal axis [74]. AFB-mediated DNA damage results in the deregulation of the cell cycle and cause HCC through the up-regulation of pro-apoptotic pathways including p53, NF-kB, BCl2, c-Myc, CDK, Ras, protein kinase C, Cyclins and CKI's [75, 76]. All these mechanisms of actions take place in the liver.

9. Conclusions

In this review, we summarize the distribution of fungi that produce aflatoxins, general properties of aflatoxins, metabolism of AFB_1 as well as the immunomodulatory effects and the mechanisms of carcinogenesis of AFB_1. All these information or data are already reported in literature.

We report from our previous study that AFB_1 inhibit the type I interferon signaling response pathway by suppressing transcript expression levels of JAK1, STAT1 and OAS3. We also report that AFB_1 suppresses the translation of STAT1 mRNA into protein. STAT1 which is a key component of the JAK–STAT-ISRE arm of the type I interferon signaling response pathway is known to exhibit its tumor suppressing function by inducing apoptosis and inhibiting angiogenesis. Therefore, by demonstrating in our study that AFB_1 inhibit translation of STAT1 mRNA into protein suggest that AFB_1 can suppress the immune system of individuals exposed to it thereby predisposing them to cancers and other diseases.

Author details

Mohamed Mutocheluh* and Patrick Williams Narkwa
Department of Clinical Microbiology, School of Medicine and Dentistry, Kwame Nkrumah University of Science and Technology, Kumasi, Ghana

*Address all correspondence to: mmutocheluh.ch@knust.edu.gh

References

[1] Blount WP. Turkey "X" disease. Journal of British Turkey Federation. 1961;**9**:52-57

[2] Sudakin DL. Dietary aflatoxin exposure and chemoprevention of cancer: A clinical review. Journal of Toxicology. Clinical Toxicology. 2003;**41**:195-204

[3] Wild CP, Gong YY. Mycotoxins and human disease: A largely ignored global health issue. Carcinogenesis. 2010;**31**:71-82

[4] IARC. Some traditional herbal medicines, some mycotoxins, naphthalene and styrene. IARC Monographs on the Evaluation of Carcinogenic Risks to Humans. Vol. 82. 2002. pp. 171-300

[5] Awuah RT, Kpodo KA. High incidence of Aspergillus flavus and aflatoxins in stored groundnut in Ghana and the use of a microbial assay to assess the inhibitory effects of plant extracts on aflatoxin synthesis. Mycopathologia. 1996;**134**(2):109-114

[6] Kpodo K, Thrane U, Hald B. Fusaria and fumonisins in maize from Ghana and their co-occurrence with aflatoxins. International Journal of Food Microbiology. 2000;**61**(2-3):147-157

[7] Oyelami O, Maxwell S, Adeoba E. Aflatoxins and ochratoxin A in the weaning food of Nigerian children Annals of tropical paediatrics. 1996;**16**(2):137-140

[8] Kumi J et al. Aflatoxins and fumonisins contamination of home-made food (weanimix) from cereal-legume blends for children. Ghana Medical Journal. 2014;**48**(3):121-126

[9] Wild CP, Hall AJ. Primary prevention of hepatocellular carcinoma in developing countries. Mutation Research - Reviews. 2000;**462**(2-3):381-393

[10] Wogan GN. Aflatoxins as risk factors for hepatocellular carcinoma in humans. Cancer Research. 1992;**52**(7 Suppl): 2114s-2118s

[11] Chen CJ, Yu MW, Liaw YF. Epidemiological characteristics and risk factors of hepatocellular carcinoma. Journal of Gastroenterology and Hepatology. 1997;**12**:S294-S308

[12] Liu Y, Wu F. Global burden of aflatoxin-induced hepatocellular carcinoma: A risk assessment. Environmental Health Perspectives. 2010;**118**:818-824

[13] Gresser I. Interferon and cancer: Therapeutic prospects Revue europeene d'etudes cliniques et biologiques. European Journal of Clinical and Biological Research. 1970;**15**:23-27

[14] Bekisz J et al. Anti-proliferative properties of type I and type II Interferon. Pharmaceuticals. 2010;**3**:994-1015

[15] Aziz TA, Aziz MA, et al. Interferon-alpha gene therapy prevents aflatoxin and carbon tetrachloride promoted hepatic carcinogenesis in rats. International Journal of Molecular Medicine. 2005;**15**(1):21-26

[16] Strosnider H et al. Workgroup report: Public health strategies for reducing aflatoxin exposure in developing countries. Environmental Health Perspectives. 2006;**114**:1989-1903

[17] Williams JH et al. Human aflatoxicosis in developing countries: A

review of toxicology, exposure, potential health consequences, and interventions. The American Journal of Clinical Nutrition. 2004;**80**(5):1106-1122

[18] Bennett JW, Kale S, Yu J. Aflatoxins: Background, toxicology and molecular biology. In: Simjee S, editor. Infectious Disease: Foodborne Diseases. Totowa, NJ, USA: Humana Press Inc.; 2007. pp. 355-373

[19] Wacoo AP, et al. Methods for detection of aflatoxins in agricultural food crops article ID 706291. 2014. p. 15

[20] Wu F et al. The health economics of aflatoxin: Global burden of disease. Aflacontrol. 2011;**4**:1-14

[21] Smela ME et al. The aflatoxin B1 formamidopyrimidine adduct plays a major role in causing the types of mutations observed in human hepatocellular carcinoma. Proceedings of the National Academy of Sciences of the United States of America. 2002;**99**:6655-6660

[22] IARC. Some Naturally Occurring Substances: Food Items and Constituents, Heterocyclic Aromatic Amines and Mycotoxins. Lyon: IARC Press; 1993

[23] Wild CP, Turner PC. The toxicology of aflatoxins as a basis for public health decisions. Mutagenesis. 2002;**17**:471-481

[24] Neal GE et al. Metabolism and toxicity of aflatoxins M1 and B1 in human-derived in vitro systems. Toxicology and Applied Pharmacology. 1998;**151**:152-158

[25] Kew, MC. Hepatocellular carcinoma. Molecular biology and genetics. In: Gastrointestinal Oncology. 2nd. ed. Kelsen DP, Daly JM, Kem SE, Levin B, Tepper JE, Van Cutsem, E. editors. 2008, Philadelphia: Lippincott: Williams and Wilkins. pp. 405-418.

[26] IARC. Aflatoxins: In overall evaluations of carcinogenicity. In: IARC Monographs on the Evaluation of the Carcinogenic Risks of Chemicals to Humans, 1987. suppl. 7. Lyon, France: International Agency for Research on Cancer. pp. 245-395

[27] NRC. Risk Assessment in the Federal Government: Managing the Process. Washington, DC: National Academy Press; 1983

[28] Gong Y et al. Aflatoxin exposure and impaired child growth in West Africa: An unexplored international public health burden? In: Leslie JF, Bandyopadhyay R, Visconti A, editors. Mycotoxins: Detection Methods, Management, Public Health and Agricultural Trade. Oxfordshire, UK: CAB International; 2008. pp. 53-65

[29] Wu, F. The global burden of disease caused by foodborne aflatoxin. WHO Commissioned Report, Foodborne Disease Burden Epidemiology Reference Group (FERG). 2010

[30] Cullen JM, Newberne PM. Acute hepatotoxicity of aflatoxins. In: Eaton DL, Groopman JD, editors. The Toxicology of Aflatoxins. New Yorke: Academic Press; 1994. pp. 3-26

[31] CDC. Outbreak of aflatoxin poisoning in eastern and central provinces, Kenya, January-July 2004 MMWR. Morbidity and Mortality Weekly Report. 2004;**53**(34):790-793

[32] Lye MS et al. An outbreak of acute hepatic encephalopathy due to severe aflatoxicosis in Malaysia. The American Journal of Tropical Medicine and Hygiene. 1995;**53**:68-72

[33] Miller DM, Wilson DM. Veterinary diseases related to aflatoxins. In: Ealton DL, Groopman JD, editors. The Toxicology of Aflatoxins: Human Health, Veterinary, and Agricultural Significance. San Diego, CA: Academic Press, Inc; 1994. pp. 347-364

[34] Hall AJ, Wild CP. Epidemiology of aflatoxin-related disease. In: Ealton DL, Groopman JD, editors. The Toxicology of Aflatoxins: Human Health, Veterinary, and Agricultural Significance. San Diego, CA: Academic Press, Inc; 1994. pp. 233-258

[35] Gong YY et al. Determinants of aflatoxin exposure in young children from Benin and Togo, West Africa: The critical role of weaning. International Journal of Epidemiology. 2003;**32**(4):556-562

[36] Gong Y, Hounsa A, Egal S. Post weaning exposure to aflatoxin results in impaired child growth: A longitudinal study in Benin. West Africa Environmental Health Perspective. 2004;**112**:1334-1338

[37] Jiang Y et al. Aflatoxin B1 albumin adduct levels and cellular immune status in Ghanaians. International Immunology. 2005;**17**(6):807-814

[38] Turner PC et al. Modification of immune function through exposure to dietary aflatoxin in Gambian children. Environmental Health Perspectives. 2003;**111**(2):217-220

[39] Jolly P, et al., Modulation of the human immune system by aflatoxin. In: Mycotoxins: Detection Methods, Management, Public Health and Agricultural Trade. Leslie JFBR, Visconti A, editors. 2008 Oxfordshire, UK: CAB International. pp. 41-52.

[40] Verma RJ. Aflatoxin cause DNA damage. International Journal of Human Genetics. 2004;**4**:231-236

[41] Bhat NK et al. Inhibition of mitochondrial protein synthesis during early stages of aflatoxin b-induced hepatocarcino-genesis. Cancer Research. 1982;**42**:1876-1880

[42] Bbosa GS et al. Aflatoxins metabolism, effects on epigenetic mechanisms and their role in carcinogenesis. Health. 2013;**5**(10A):14-34

[43] Eaton DL, Gallagher EP. Mechanisms of aflatoxin carcinogenesis. Annual Review of Pharmacology and Toxicology. 1994;**34**:135-172

[44] Bbosa GS et al. Re-view of the biological and health effects of aflatoxins on body organs and body systems. In: Aflatoxins-Recent Advances and Future Prospects. Vol. 12. London: Intechopen Publisher; 2013. pp. 239-265

[45] Bruneau JC et al. Aflatoxins B1, B2 and G1 modulate cytokine secretion and cell surface marker expression in J774A. 1 murine macrophages. Toxicology In Vitro. 2012;**26**:686-693

[46] Dugyala RR, Sharma RP. The effect of aflatoxin B1 on cytokine mRNA and corresponding protein levels in peritoneal macrophages and splenic lymphocytes. International Journal of Immunopharmacology. 1996;**18**:599-608

[47] Marin D et al. Changes in performance, blood parameters, humoral and cellular immune responses in weanling piglets exposed to low doses of aflatoxin. Journal of Animal Science. 2002;**80**:1250-1257

[48] Li Y et al. Effects of lipoic acid on immune function, the antioxidant defense system, and inflammation-related genes expression of broiler chickens fed aflatoxin contaminated

diets. International Journal of Molecular Sciences. 2014;**15**:5649-5662

[49] Qian G et al. Aflatoxin B1 modulates the expression of phenotypic markers and cytokines by splenic lymphocytes of male F344 rats. Journal of Applied Toxicology. 2014;**34**:241-249

[50] Forouharmehr A, Harkinezhad T, Qasemi-Panahi B. Evaluation of STAT5A gene expression in aflatoxin B1 treated bovine mammary epithelial cells. Advanced Pharmaceutical Bulletin. 2013;**3**(2):461-464

[51] Rossano F et al. Secondary metabolites of Aspergillus exert immunobiological effects on human monocytes. Research in Microbiology. 1999;**150**:13-19

[52] Hahon N, Booth JA, Stewart JD. Aflatoxin inhibition of viral interferon induction. Antimicrobial Agents and Chemotherapy. 1979;**16**(3):277-282

[53] Narkwa PW, Blackbourn DJ, Mutocheluh M. Aflatoxin B1 inhibits the type 1 interferon response pathway via STAT1 suggesting another mechanism of hepatocellular carcinoma. Infectious Agents and Cancer. 2017;**12**:17

[54] Rasooly R, Hernlem B, Friedman M. Low levels of aflatoxin B1, ricin, and milk enhance recombinant protein production in mammalian cells. PLoS One. 2013;**8**(8):e71682

[55] Dunn GP, Koebel CM, Schreiber RD. Interferons, immunity and cancer immunoediting. Nature Reviews. Immunology. 2006;**6**:836-848

[56] Khodarev NN, Roizman B, Weichselbaum RR. Molecular pathways: interferon/stat1 pathway: Role in the tumor resistance to genotoxic stress and aggressive growth. Clinical Cancer Research. 2012;**18**(11):3015-3021

[57] Pensa S et al. STAT1 and STAT3 in tumorigenesis: Two sides of the same coin. In: Stephanou A, editor. JAK-STAT Pathway in Disease. Austin: Landes Bioscience; 2008. pp. 100-121

[58] Fadelu T, Rebbeck TR. The rising burden of cancer in low- and middle-Human Development Index countries. Cancer. 2021;**127**(16):2864-2866

[59] Bulatao-Jayme J et al. A case-control dietary study of primary liver cancer risk from aflatoxin exposure. International Journal of Epidemiology. 1982;**11**(2):112-119

[60] Van Rensburg S et al. Hepatocellular carcinoma and dietary aflatoxin in Mozambique and Transkei. British Journal of Cancer. 1985;**51**:713-726

[61] Yeh FS et al. Hepatitis B virus, aflatoxins, and hepatocellular carcinoma in southern Guangxi, China. Cancer Research. 1989;**49**(9):2506-2509

[62] Mace K et al. Aflatoxin B1-induced DNA adduct formation and p53 mutations in CYP450-expressing human liver cell lines. Carcinogenesis. 1997;**18**(7):1291-1297

[63] Gallagher EP et al. Role of human microsomal and human complementary DNA-expressed cytochromes P4501A2 and P4503A4 in the bioactivation of aflatoxin B1. Cancer Research. 1994;**54**:101-108

[64] Waters R et al. The repair of large DNA adducts in mammalian cells. Mutation Research. 1992;**273**:145-155

[65] Sarasin AR, Smith CA, Hanawalt PC. Repair of DNA in human cells after

treatment with activated aflatoxin B1. Cancer Research. 1977;**37**:1786-1793

[66] Hsu IC et al. Mutational hotspot in the p53 gene in human hepatocellular carcinomas. Nature. 1991;**350**:427-428

[67] Aguilar F, Hussain SP, Cerutti P. Aflatoxin B1 induces the transversion of G→T in codon 249 of the p53 tumor suppressor gene in human hepatocytes. Proceedings of the National Academy of Sciences of the United States of America. 1993;**90**:8586-8590

[68] Martin J, Dufour JF. Tumor suppressor and hepatocellular carcinoma. World Journal of Gastroenterology. 2008;**14**:1720-1733

[69] Bressac B et al. Selective G to T mutations of p53 gene in hepatocellular carcinoma from southern Africa. Nature. 1991;**350**:429-431

[70] Ozturk M. p53 mutation in hepatocellular carcinoma after aflatoxin exposure. Lancet. 1991;**338**:1356-1359

[71] Lereau M et al. Interactions between hepatitis B virus and aflatoxin B1: Effects on p53 induction in HepaRG cells. Journal of General Virology. 2012;**93**:640-650

[72] Hollstein M, Hainaut P. Massively regulated genes: The example of TP53. The Journal of Pathology. 2010;**220**:164-173

[73] Zhu L et al. miR-34a screened by miRNA profiling negatively regulates Wnt/β-catenin signaling pathway in Aflatoxin B1 induced hepatotoxicity. Scientific Reports. 2015;**5**:16732

[74] Ubagai T et al. Aflatoxin B1 modulates the insulin-like growth factor-2 dependent signaling axis. Toxicology In Vitro. 2010;**24**:783-789

[75] Dai Y et al. Aflatoxin B1-induced epigenetic alterations: An overview. Food and Chemical Toxicology. 2017;**109**(1):683-689

[76] Rieswijk L et al. Aflatoxin B1 induces persistent epigenomic effects in primary human hepatocytes associated with hepatocellular carcinoma. Toxicology. 2016;**350-352**:31-39